Sneaky Parenting

Sneaky Parenting

Smart shortcuts to happy families

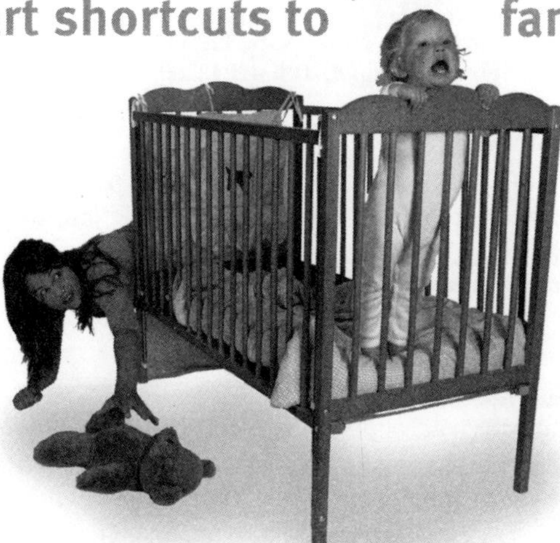

Jo Wiltshire

Editor Roni Jay

Viva Books

New Delhi | Mumbai | Chennai | Kolkata | Bangalore | Hyderabad | Kochi | Guwahati

First Indian Edition 2010

VIVA BOOKS PRIVATE LIMITED

- 4737/23 Ansari Road, Daryaganj, New Delhi 110 002
  E-mail: vivadelhi@vivagroupindia.net, Tel. 42242200
- 76, Service Industries, Shirvane, Sector 1, Nerul, Navi Mumbai 400 706
  E-mail: vivamumbai@vivagroupindia.net, Tel. 27721273, 27721274
- Jamals Fazal Chambers, 26 Greams Road, Chennai 600 006
  E-mail: vivachennai@vivagroupindia.net, Tel. 28290304, 28294241
- B-103, Jindal Towers, 21/1A/3 Darga Road, Kolkata 700 017
  E-mail: vivakolkata@vivagroupindia.net, Tel. 22836381, 22816713
- 7, Sovereign Park Apartments, 56-58, K. R. Road, Basavanagudi, Bangalore 560 004
  E-mail: vivabangalore@vivagroupindia.net, Tel. 26607409, 26607410
- 101-102 Mughal Marc Apartments, 3-4-637 to 641, Narayanguda, Hyderabad 500 029
  E-mail: vivahyderabad@vivagroupindia.net, Tel. 27564481, 27564482
- Beevi Towers, First Floor, SRM Road, Kaloor, Kochi 682 018, Kerala
  E-mail: vivakochi@vivagroupindia.net, Tel: 0484-2403055, 2403056
- 232, GNB Road, Beside UCO Bank, Silpukhuri, Guwahati 781 003
  E-mail: vivaguwahati@vivagroupindia.net, Tel: 0361-2666386

www.vivagroupindia.com

Published by arrangement with

Crimson Publishing,
a division of Crimson Business Ltd
Westminster House, Kew Road
Richmond, Surrey TW9 2ND

ISBN : 978-81-309-1483-1

Published by Vinod Vasishtha for Viva Books Private Limited, 4737/23, Ansari Road, Daryaganj, New Delhi - 110 002.

Printed and bound by Raj Press, R-3, Inderpuri, New Delhi - 110 012.

Contents

Introduction

This book is aimed at parents who wish they could cook like Annabel Karmel, timetable like Gina Ford and listen like Penelope Leach, but who, just sometimes, can only manage baked beans, botched bedtimes and bribery.

This is not a book which tells you it's OK to be a terrible mother/father – 'sneaky' it may be, and hopefully with lots of useful shortcuts – but safe, caring and loving always. This is a book aimed at getting you from first steps to starting school armed with mothers' and fathers' top tips on doing the best for your child without the guilt trip that seems to come as standard for today's 'have it all' parent.

Forget Yummy Mummies with washboard stomachs and surgically-attached Mouli mills – today's real parents need instant inspiration. You haven't cooked a batch of freshly-puréed root vegetables? Then which of your freezer food is the best nutritional option for your hungry child? You're stuck on the M5 in a traffic jam with two bored and vocal children? What inspiration can you pull out of the hat?

Every parent knows the books they 'ought' to be reading. From the classic child-rearing manuals to modern tomes on baby whispering/yoga/massage/growing-your-own-genius, they demand a lifelong subscription to the Perfect Parent Club which leaves most people feeling incompetent, stressed and guilty as hell for not coming up to scratch.

I think that parents have enough theory pushed at them. This book contains advice from the front line. It is packed with tips and anecdotes from real parents who have seen, done and dealt with it all.

It is an unapologetically subjective look at modern parenting for the conscientious but overstretched parent. It's not a how-to manual – just a fact-packed and inspirational exploration of realistic ways to make your child's toddler years – and your time together – fun (and as stress-free as life with a mini-dictator can get).

As for me, I have a four year old daughter Evie, who is my anecdotal source and inspiration. She, her friends, cousins and a host of other children will hopefully cover the gamut of childhood challenges you might come across. Evie's little brother Charlie has also arrived now, just in time to contribute to the 'preparing for a new sibling' topic.

From picky eaters to prima donnas, from chicken nugget addicts to soggy potty-refusers, from buggy battlers to bedtime hell-raisers – this is the book which accepts your little darlings in all their Technicolor splendour and tells you how to deal with the real stuff – quickly, with humour and in time for a cup of tea with EastEnders.

Good luck!

Jo Wiltshire

CHAPTER 1

Sleep

Bedtime without the blues; from cot to bed without the walkabout

It's one of the things we ponder with trepidation when we're expecting a baby, and a major preoccupation of those of us with newborns. In fact, it remains an issue for many of us until our children become teenagers and magically transform into creatures which rarely emerge from the murky fug of their duvets. Will they sleep? *Please*, let them go to sleep.

If one thing leaves parents reeling between feelings of despair, fury, incomprehension and a state of wanting to quietly burrow a tunnel under the carpet and stay there, it's the issue of their child's slumber. So it seems a good place to start this book.

It doesn't matter if the child in question is five weeks old or five years; if they are a bad sleeper, they hold their whole family to ransom. Sleep worries have one major factor which distinguishes them from most other child-rearing problems, which is that this is the one area which directly affects you and your abilities to cope too.

If a child won't eat their greens, you have strategies. You can hide vegetables in a sauce, or give them some fruit instead. And you get to eat your own tea as heartily as ever. But if a child won't sleep, that's it. For the child, and for you too. They cry, you chew the duvet. You simply drew the short straw in the sleep lottery.

At least, that's what it can feel like. Especially during one of those conversations with other parents when one says the inevitable line: "Of course, I've been so lucky with little Nancy … she just loves her sleep. Two naps a day while I nip round with the vacuum cleaner/file a company report/bake a cake, and still in bed like clockwork at 7pm for 12 hours straight."

Meanwhile, you're facing a 10-minute nap once every other day but only if you drive round the block until they nod off, followed by bed at 11pm and waking every 40 minutes until you get up again at six.

You despair. So you look for help. And there's plenty on offer – for this is where the Big Gun Gurus really gear up for action. 'Sleep training!' screams one. 'Absolute routine!' confirms another. 'Family bed, cuddles on demand!' offers yet another. You choose one, feeling inadequate if you can't follow their advice to the letter, and end up not just tired but demoralised to boot.

"Ah, it must be so hard," tuts the Perfect Sleeper's mother in gleeful sympathy. "I suppose some babies are good sleepers, and some (looking at yours) just … aren't. Nothing you can do about it."

Rubbish. Let's get this straight from the start. Yes, some children sleep better than others. Fact. But you are not a powerless observer of your child. You *can* influence this.

If you think, however, that you're going to pick up one single book which contains the key to everlasting sleep nirvana overnight, you're wrong. Your child is an individual, and you have to find out which buttons to press. But there are lots of fantastic buttons, so read on.

Priorities

Firstly, know what your aim is. What is most important – a nap in the day? Or a proper evening to yourself? Or a later bedtime, but all sleeping together in the same bed? Take off your rose-tinted specs here – do what you really want, not what some expert tells you is best.

Then, know your child. Take a good hard look at their likes, dislikes and triggers, sleeping-wise. "Heather, now three, was an excellent sleeper who required no 'sleep training' whatsoever, slept 7pm-7am and still does," says Caroline, whose daughter is now four. "I adopted the opinion that any child could be a good sleeper if the parents wanted it badly enough. I was very opinionated regarding people who rocked their babies to sleep, fed them in the night when they didn't need it, and – the ultimate sin – took their babies to bed with them.

"Then along came Murray. There is no sleep-related baby book or technique I haven't tried. At eight months, on average, he woke at least two nights a week every 40 minutes from midnight until the morning. I have learned to accept and appreciate any sleep I may get in a night, instead of cursing him that I have been up six times or more getting stressed and frustrated. We go to bed about 9pm to get three hours' sleep before midnight."

You will find everyone has an opinion. When they move on to solids they'll sleep through, they say. When they start to move about, to walk, go to nursery … but in the meantime, it's up to you to find compromises.

"From birth, Murray refused to sleep on his back," says Caroline. "I tried every trick in the book, and no matter what I did, he would always end up face down, lying on his hands. Now, we let him. I believe that had I let him do this earlier, I would not be in the mess I'm in now."

Jo, mother of Archie, four, and Charlotte, two, agrees that too much interference, however loving, can work against you. "With your first child, you just want to watch them fall asleep as if they can't do it without your help," she says. "You sing to them, feed them, rock them, stroke their face, shake noisy toys and wonder why you are still there after an hour or more. What you should do is sleep training. At about 12 weeks we did this for Archie and it only took a couple of nights.

"The second child is much easier to deal with. You haven't got the time to spend helping them go to sleep so they learn much quicker to do it on their own."

A general consensus of good tips from parents I have asked includes the following (but do discard – without a guilt trip – any individual ones which do not work for you):

- Put the baby down before it is asleep, so it does not get used to relying on your cuddles/rocking/singing.
- Keep a general routine when convenient – bath, feed, bed – but don't let it become a straitjacket. Make the odd exception (such as on family occasions) so the baby is adaptable.
- Don't tiptoe around – you'll be making a rod for your own back. "Keep a low drone in the background – the vacuum cleaner, the TV, the washing machine," says Evie's grandmother, Annie. "If you already have a child who demands total silence, start the drone off at a very low level and up it gradually over a number of days." You might even consider making a tape recording of "white noise" such as a washing machine, and playing it in the child's room. Apparently you can also buy these.
- Blackout blinds. I love these so much I've even put some in our room. Evie's blinds make her sleep later, and go to bed easier on light summer nights. If we're on holiday and there are no blinds, she sleeps a noticeably shorter night.
- Dummies. If you use them, don't scrimp – put several in the cot so one can be 'found' easily in the night without your help.
- A comforter, blankie or teddy. Best tip – choose it yourself, before they're even born. You can put anything in their Moses basket or crib before they're six months old and they'll attach to it. So choose something washable, replaceable and not too big, before they opt for your nas-

tiest tea towel or most mangy muslin instead. Get two or three so you can keep swapping and washing them, or they'll hate the clean ones and always cry for the stinky grubby one.

- For twins, a certain steeliness is required. Jane, mother of twins Ethan and Hannah, two, as well as big sister Emily, five, says: "At night, if one baby wakes up for a feed, always wake the other one at the same time. I would feed one baby and my husband the other. The idea is that they will feed at the same time and roughly settle at the same time so you're not losing out on any more sleep than if you had a 'singleton'. If you're on your own, leave it 20–25 minutes before waking the second twin. You can't afford to have a baby at your breast or bottle for an hour or more when you have two."
- Georgia, mother of twins Holly and Callum, one, as well as big brother Woody, four, suggests taking shifts to fit sleep in around twins while they are still babies and feeding at night. "Ed and I split every night – Ed would do from 9pm to 2am while I slept, and I would do 2am to 7am while he slept. You could do the same for single babies too. It meant that we both got five hours a night, which is a luxury with twins."
- "Use a red light bulb, or a 12w night bulb, so that you don't startle the baby awake when you go in for feeds and checks," says Jake, father of Milly, one.
- Some swear by baby sleeping bags – Evie loved them. No covers to get tangled in, no cold feet. But others disagree:

"Someone told me Murray would stay on his back if I put him in a sleeping bag and tucked it into the base of the cot," says Caroline. "He was uncomfortable. It just made the situation worse."

- An extra sheet, or a pillowcase, put over the top half of the cot mattress. "Sicky messes can be whipped away and a clean sheet is there waiting," says Annie.
- Your nightie or unwashed T-shirt – preferably smelling of milk – in the cot with the baby. Some swear this helps them to settle.
- For an overly-tired or stimulated baby, a 'white-out' – put the baby to your shoulder and face them to a white wall. This relaxes the baby and makes them sleepy. "You can hang a white muslin over a baby car seat or carry cot if you're out," says Jess, whose daughter is now four. "Molly would fall asleep beautifully for a nap if I did this."
- Static Moses baskets and cribs. "Be aware that with rocking ones, when the startle reflex happens, it then rocks the basket and wakes them up," says Caroline. "Buy one that has a fixed position too."
- Swings. "When I needed to work at home the battery–operated swing was my saviour," says Jo. "It was one of the best items we bought and I wish we'd had it sooner."
- Get your partner, if you have one, to do all the night-time attendances. "Make sure he is sleeping closest to the door and you can sleep through it," says Jo.

- And on moving from the basket to the cot: "I worried so much about the transition, I spent hours winding the sheets through the cot bars to make it more cosy," says Jess. "As it turned out, neither of mine were remotely bothered – so I suppose my tip there would be not to worry too much in advance."

Big bed battles

At some point, you and your baby will reach a compromise between what is desirable, sleep-wise, and what is realistic for that child. Things will potter haphazardly along these lines for a while … until they outgrow the cot.

And then, here you go again.

Older toddlers and pre-schoolers bring with them a whole new catalogue of sleep challenges. The nappy/wet bed ones are dealt with in the potty training section. The rest tend to fall into two categories: keeping them in the bed/bedroom, and persuading them that 5am is not a good time for breakfast.

Keeping them there involves a similar kind of 'firm but controlled' approach that getting them to sleep in a cot did.

First, set the scene. Talk about 'Big Girl rooms' and 'Big Boy rooms'. Let them get excited about acquiring a new bed, and allow them to pick out a few new furnishings.

Consider a toddler bed rather than a full-sized single – less economical, perhaps, but much cosier for a little person. And maybe keep the cot *and* the bed in the room for a week or so, so they appear to have the 'choice' between the two. I tried this with Evie, who banished the cot after two nights and never looked back.

Also, if a child is moving out of a cot to make way for a new sibling, make the move well in advance. "We moved Archie because Charlotte was coming, when he was just over two," says Jo. "We did it well before she arrived, so it wasn't 'his' cot any more – he wasn't forced out because she needed it."

Make the new, grown-up room appealing. Novelty racing car beds or fairy canopies, for larger budgets; colourful rugs and a new lamp for smaller ones.

Accessories which also give off light are a good way to avoid the night-time frights. Fairy lights (use the safe, cool-to-touch ones for children) can make a room into a comforting grotto. Glow-in-the-dark stars on the ceiling give would-be mini astronauts something to gaze at.

"We let Ben have one of those back-lit fish tanks on a chest of drawers in his room," says Ben's father David, whose son is now four. "He loved the main light going off at bedtime."

Older children might be trusted with a child's torch. If not, there are some very unusual nightlights about. "We conditioned Molly to associate her musical aquarium nightlight with going to sleep from quite an early age," says Jess. "It always played the same lullaby as she dropped off, then when she woke in the night at first we turned it on for her, but when she got a bit older she would turn it on herself and go back to sleep."

When it comes to actually shutting the door and leaving them, be firm. If there are two of you, present a united front. Switch which one of you 'does' bedtime, to prevent clinginess.

"Make sure they are wearing plenty of bedtime clothes to allow for the covers falling off," says Jo. "Archie wears socks all year round. And don't fall for a guilt trip – at three-and-a-half he used to beg me to lie with him until he fell asleep. Having a cuddle is a lovely thing, but it doesn't help them. He'd wake up when I'd gone and cry out for me again – and I was so tired I'd often fall asleep with him. He now goes to sleep alone, but with the door open, and night lights guiding the way to the toilet."

A nervous child needs comfort, while retaining their independence. "We recorded ourselves reading some of Esme's favourite stories and would then play these back at low volume for her after we'd left the room," says three year old Esme's father Peter. "We also swapped round her baby monitor ends, so she could hear us moving about and talking downstairs, and knew we were there."

For children who protest they are not sleepy, try a little lavender oil on a hanky near their pillow, or you can buy lavender-stuffed cuddly toys that can be microwaved to make them warm and smelly.

"I would also say, for a pre-schooler, to avoid long daytime naps," says Alice, whose son is four. 'Sam will settle beautifully if he has been awake all day, but if he has had even a 10-minute cat-nap in the car, he will struggle to settle until much, much later and say 'I'm just not tired, Mummy'."

Annie, who perfected this technique on me and still uses it with my daughter Evie, also recommends visualisation. "We would cuddle quietly and make up a scene in our heads," she remembers. "You would add things you could see, like 'a bird sitting on a tree' or 'a fairy by the lake'. Eventually you would just nod off."

For those who are bothered by night-time 'monsters', a little imagination can work wonders in counteracting their fears. "Heather had a monster in her ear that would come out at night," remembers Caroline. "Now I don't know where it came from, but that wee thing stayed there for about six months. We ended up having to pull the monster out of her ear each night and throw him out of the window. The garden monster (friendly chap) who guarded the house at night to stop any bad monsters getting in would then send him packing."

Twins can present their own particular problems when it comes to big beds – egging each other on to get out of them, for a start. Jane, mother of Ethan and Hannah, says: "Some mothers of twins swear by keeping them in the same room – but I gave in after two sleep-deprived nights and put them in separate rooms. If you want any time to yourself, you have to be firm at bedtime and set the ground rules straight away. With twins, a routine is essential."

And for children who fancy themselves as escape artists, I have had a couple of rather extreme tips: a bolt on the outside of the door, and olive oil on the door handle. Depending on your nerve, possibly a better approach might be firm but repeated repositioning back in the bed.

Early birds

Once the child is firmly tucked up and sleeping peacefully, the next problem occurs in the morning when they want to get up, and you don't. "Is it Up Time yet Mummy?" is Evie's current refrain, yelled at a volume to wake half the street.

top tips

Best tips include:

- One of those light timers designed to turn your lamps on to prevent burglaries. Set it to 7am, and set the rule that they don't get out of bed until the lamp goes on. If they wake before, they can play or read quietly. Sneaky parents can set it for later at weekends.

- A radio alarm clock set for the chosen time. "Unbelievable!" says Jess. "Molly was getting us up any time from 5.30am, but now she understands that it isn't morning, and she can't get up, until the music plays. I recommend Radio 2 and set the alarm for just before 7am so she gets music and not the news bulletin. It really works – some mornings you can hear her muttering to herself: 'Come on music, come on!'"

Finally, remember you're not alone. All parents want more sleep. Your children will not sleep enough to match your requirements until they hit 13 and are genetically programmed not to emerge from their rooms for days at a time. Until that time, sleep when they do, nap when you can, draw up some basic rules, and use any trick available to you.

CHAPTER 2

Food

What's quick but still good for them – and how to deal with fussy eaters and vegetable haters

Food – another biggie, and another good place to start getting sneaky, since we worry about what we're putting into our children from Day One. Are they getting enough? Does it make the grade nutritionally? Are they on the right weight percentile on the chart? Have they made friends with fruit and veg yet? Have we poured enough of our hearts and souls into our home-made batch cooking to alleviate that niggling doubt that we might somehow, on the food front, be … lacking?

Food both unites and levels all parents. It doesn't matter if your child is a violin genius or a mini-hoodlum, if they are potty trained at six months or six years, neatly starched or dressed top to toe in wrinkled rags – if they're staging a sit-in over a carrot, all parents feel that same sense of utter frustration, worry and despair.

So if we're going to win the food war with our children, it seems, we're going to have to get clever. Rule One – it's not actually a war. Really, it doesn't have to be. If you don't think it is, they won't either. And Rule Two – 'convenient' doesn't have to mean 'nasty'. It just means convenient. For you. And if it's good but convenient, you're more likely to keep it up than if you embark upon an edifying but near-on impossible quest to feed your child lengthy, cook-from-scratch recipes fit for a king day after day.

Obviously, a home-cooked concoction festooned with perky steamed vegetables is preferable to the ubiquitous bullet-like chicken nuggets and chips; we all know this. And most of the time, most of us manage an all-round healthy diet that gives our children the best start in life.

But just occasionally, life gets in the way. It's tea time, you've just got in, and your Delia skills have been caught short. You need nutritious food in five minutes flat – and no guilty conscience.

Essentials

Don't panic – most kitchen cupboards, with just the odd helping hand from a local village shop or corner store, are a mine of quick but good food.

It helps if you keep a few emergency supplies. "Fruit is instant and delicious – bananas are a godsend," says Dave, father of Joshua, eight, Arthur, five, and Mabel, three. "Other favourite stand-bys in our house include:

- Eggs (boiled with soldiers will engage most young children, who love to dunk).
- Baked beans (excellent with a microwaved jacket potato and a sprinkling of cheese).

- Decent ham – not the wafer-thin, practically all-water kind (can be put on sliced bread with a little cheese and some sliced tomatoes and mushrooms and grilled for two-minute pizzas)."

Even the foods that make supercilious mothers turn up their noses can, if bought carefully, be decent emergency options. Ketchup can be the organic kind and is actually full of antioxidants; most supermarkets do breaded chicken that is 100 per cent breast meat and organic; frozen vegetables are actually fresher and contain more nutrients than less-than-pristine fresh versions.

Yes, that's right, freezers are not evil. "Don't automatically assume frozen means bad," says Annie, grandmother of Evie. "Fish fingers – breaded, not battered – if used sparingly are a great way to get children to eat fish."

Start as you mean to go on – it's never too early to use a few tricks to get good healthy food into your child. Babies, for example, will love an ice lolly made from breast milk or formula milk rather than sugary bright pink chemicals – especially when they're teething. "You can buy little lolly-making kits with sticks and plastic moulds," says Marianne, mother of Milly, one. "You just pour some expressed milk or formula into the mould and stick it in the freezer. They're small, so they're usually really quick to freeze."

In the early days, if you do manage to cook a lengthy family meal – or are simply in the mood for a spot of batch cooking – think forward. "Pound shops do small plastic lidded pots that take a mini meal-sized portion of food each and which make a great healthy ready-meal from the freezer for little ones," says Steve, father of Lily, two. "They're also good for dads who want an easy-to-prepare tea." No E-numbers, preservatives or strange thickening agents, but all ready at the ding of a microwave. Perfect.

Jane, mother of twins Ethan and Hannah, two, and big sister Emily, five, adapts this for twin feeding. "Double all your recipes, purée and freeze in ice cube trays to start, or in bigger portions later on," she says. "Whatever you can do in advance helps with the day-to-day care of twins."

We're not talking food preparation on an earth mother-inspired industrial scale here. For babies, purée everything you eat that's not overly spicy. As they get more used to food, leave it a little lumpy to encourage them to try new textures. For young toddlers, just ladle a little of whatever you are having into a pot – complete with leftover veggies, if you have any. For older preschoolers, cook double quantities of whatever they're having for tea, and freeze half. Bolognaise sauce is perfect for this – it can be defrosted and poured over something appealing like pasta wheels (boys love these) in minutes. It can also hide a multitude of otherwise-spurned vegetables.

top tips

Ah yes, vegetables. And fruit. The major challenges. This is where you have to get creative. Good sneaky tips include:

- A mild chilli with baked beans instead of kidney beans to make it more palatable.
- A sprinkle of cinnamon on veggies to add sweetness without empty calories.

- Tangerine, clementine or satsuma segments broken up and frozen for tasty summer treats. "Milly loves these more than ice cream," says Jake.
- Fruit kebabs – banana segments, apple and orange bits and berries on a blunt stick.
- Orange juice used sparingly stirred into a hot savoury meal. "This cools it down and adds a bit of sweetness," says Steve.
- Jellies made with fruit juice or with pureed fruits and vegetables. "Why buy the E-number-filled versions?" asks Jake.
- Yoghurt-coated dried fruit from health shops presented as treats instead of sweets (Evie now prefers these to the real thing).
- Diced veg added to a shop-bought jar of ragu sauce (if you have no time to make your own).

Think different

Remember, fresh doesn't mean difficult. Smoothies make a fun and pretty instant protein shot for either breakfast or at tea time – just liquidise soya or cow's milk and banana with whatever you have in: yoghurt, tofu, soft fruits, peanut butter, honey, wheat germ. "Stick it in a glass or cup with a wide straw, and it's a treat for children of any age – and as filling and nutritious as a traditional meal," says Dave. "Josh will have the peanut butter version for breakfast as often as he's allowed it."

Often, it's all in the presentation. Make it fun. "Use big bowls for pasta and 'wet' meals," says David, father of Ben, four. "Not only can he pick the food up better, but he likes eating with a big spoon."

Know your child – some children will find spaghetti chopped into short lengths much easier, while some will be so engaged with 'sucking up' the long lengths that they'll have eaten more than they realised.

If they're not keen on something, adapt it. "We sometimes make tea a 'carpet picnic' as a treat," says David. "We use those cardboard lunch boxes you get in child-friendly cafes. And when Ben went through a stage of not liking to drink milk, we used to give him a straw to dip in his cereal bowl, and he'd finish the lot."

Be flexible. A combination that might seem disgusting to you is fine if it helps your child accept nutritious food. If they love raisins, and will eat a fish pie as long as it's got raisins in it, so be it.

And don't be afraid to bend the truth sometimes. I wanted Evie to eat dried cranberries at a time when she was suffering from cystitis. She adamantly refused. But when she saw them in a bowl, she said: "Are these sultanas?" When I mumbled an indistinct "Hmmm," she ate the lot.

Fussy tactics

Fussy eaters can drive parents to distraction. The best tip is not to make it a battle. For fussier children – especially older ones who are yearning to express their own tastes – why not let them mix their own meals occasionally? Breakfast is perfect for this. Use half a dozen old yoghurt pots, fill them with a selection of foods such as oats, sugar-free cereals, chopped fruits such as apples and bananas, dried fruits such as raisins and apricots, seeds such as sunflower and pumpkin, and some natural yoghurt – and then let them choose what they want, mix it into their own bowl and add the milk (a small amount, pre-measured). This is healthy, takes very little preparation, but engages a child brilliantly well when you're trying to iron that shirt for work.

Other fussy-eater tactics are:

- "Giving a child choice can work wonders," says Annie. "But don't make it an open choice. Don't say "Would you like peas with that?" because the answer will invariably be no. Say "Would you like peas or beans? Or both? But you have to choose one.""
- Apply a little social pressure. "Ask one of their friends round for tea," says Annie. "It's amazing that kids will eat all sorts of things at other people's houses that they won't at home. Equally, another child will eat what you put in front of them in your house. And if your child sees them eating it, they may well give it a go too. Even broccoli."
- Caroline, mother of Heather, four, who was difficult to wean and still takes little interest in food, has found imagination is the key. "Bran flakes in our house are served as 'crisps' in a bowl without milk – they get taken out of resealable freezer bags," she says. "Right now, we pretend to be animals. I tell her that the animal she wants to be eats

the food in question – quite often she is a dog, so I tell her dogs eat haggis (we're Scottish), or she is a penguin and penguins eat fish fingers."

- It can help to relate food to a favourite film or television programme. "Heather pretends to be Bruce the shark in *Finding Nemo* – she will eat lemon sole or trout this way."
- Caroline also uses role-play around cafés and waitressing, with Heather as the customer and Caroline serving tea on Heather's toy tea set. "It's amazing what she will try that she wouldn't normally eat."
- And participation is also important. "Heather helps wash the veggies and cut them up – if she has ownership over what we are having, she will maybe give them a try. The 'Daddy I've made tea for you' trick works a treat. She also helps with shopping lists and paying at the checkout when we're shopping."
- With twins, fussiness is doubly frustrating. Jane says: "After several months of doing various different meals for Hannah and Ethan, I realised this was crazy – actually, the health visitor realised this was crazy – so now I cook one meal and that's that. Especially if you have other children as well, you can't be cooking more meals than the school dinner lady."

Hands on

Participation is a key thing even for good eaters. I know not every family these days can gather round the table at teatime like The Waltons, but if an opportunity presents itself to eat together, grab it.

Rediscover your inner child – 'nursery food' is great for all the family. Think scrambled eggs, baked potatoes with cheese, sandwiches. Let the children help make them and set them out on plastic plates.

Let your child help you prepare a 'meat and veg' foil pocket à la Jamie Oliver – just pop in some chicken breast, chopped up veggies and a spoonful of stock into a folded piece of foil and stick it in the oven for about 20 minutes to half an hour until the juices run clear. It's great to unwrap and see the whole meal waiting for you.

Or make your own pizzas – just buy the bases, then have fun chopping up lots of fresh toppings and allow your child to choose which favourites go on each family member's pizza.

Eating out

A final word on food – don't let all your efforts cease the moment you step outside your front door. In fact, eating while out and about can be even more of a challenge – and it's easy to think that, in the same way dieters think food from their partner's plate doesn't contain calories, food eaten outside the home doesn't have to 'matter'. The odd trip to a fast food joint is fine. But, if you can brave the guerrilla warfare techniques your little one will employ as you approach the counter, there are ways to make the experience a little less artery-clogging.

top tips

With burger restaurants, the following tips might help:

- Ditch the sauces, dressings and mayonnaise.
- Ask for juice, water or milk instead of fizzy drinks with children's meals.
- A simple hamburger is much better than nuggets or fried chicken or onion rings.
- If they have to have fries, order a small portion.
- Consider taking a freezer bag of baby carrots, chopped veg or fruit such as grapes to supplement the main meal and replace chips. "We've always done this, and Josh still eats the chopped carrots even now he's eight," says Paul, whose children are eight, five and three. "For Arthur and Mabel, it's the norm. They don't even question it."

Often, a child will enjoy going to a tea shop or café more than to a fast food restaurant – especially the younger ones who haven't discovered the "plastic toy" enticement yet. And here, you can find great child–friendly food:

- Baked potatoes (Evie's favourite. Even when a child is very young, they will eat the innards scooped out and mashed with butter and beans)
- Wholewheat rolls
- Grilled chicken or fish sandwiches
- Soup

If it's a grown-up restaurant, most will do a simple bowl of pasta with tomato sauce, or you can mix and match from the adults' dishes to create a child-friendly version on an extra plate.

And remember – if you go out armed with snacks, you won't have to make emergency stops in nasty fried food palaces. Children usually love a little Tupperware box filled with healthy snacks which they can hold in their car seats while travelling. And if it's a long journey, soup is great – put it in a flask, not too hot. They love the idea of making a road–side stop and drinking it from a cup.

The trick with all of this is confidence. Most children eat what they require – and have differing needs and appetites. If a generally healthy child goes off something, or will only eat one type of food for a few days, it won't matter in the long run.

Be aware – the vehemence with which a child refuses to eat something increases in direct proportion to the amount of blood, sweat and tears you have put into it. Be prepared for this – don't take it personally. Just because you grew the carrot, peeled it tenderly and sautéed it in the finest virgin olive oil, doesn't mean your child will overcome a lifelong distaste for carrots overnight. Don't let food become a battleground – either between you and your child, or you and the opinionated world-at-large. Forget the food fascists – as long as a diet is varied and imaginative at best, and simple and fresh at a grab, your child won't go far wrong.

CHAPTER 3

Health

Bruises and scrapes, sniffs and coughs, teething and tears – tips for the small stuff

To start with, I am not a doctor. Neither am I some kind of medicine woman with a handful of Mother Nature's magic miracles up my sleeve. I have, let me admit, done my fair share of pestering doctors and their receptionists, as well as the trusty NHS Direct hotline, with tremulous queries and worries.

In short, I don't know any more than you do regarding children's health – just maybe a little more regarding my own children's particular weaknesses and foibles. And writing about health is a rather hefty responsibility.

So, just to be completely clear, please don't treat this chapter as any kind of bible or prescription regarding your own child's health. This is a chapter devoted to what I would call everyday complaints, those constant niggles that accompany any young child's daily life – from nappy rash and teething, colds and coughs to bruised knees and common childhood illnesses.

If your child has a high or persistent fever, is limp, listless, inconsolable or drooling, or has convulsions, a rash, a stiff neck or bloody mucus, call a doctor. If they are difficult to rouse, call a doctor. If they don't have these specific symptoms but they are poorly and just simply not themselves, or if you have a gut feeling that something is badly wrong, call a doctor. You know your child. And nobody will mind if it turns out to be a false alarm.

Other than that, though, everyday health is a preoccupation with most parents, and most will have favourite sneaky tips up their sleeves to deal with it. From those first days of cradle cap and spotty noses to the delights of pre-school nit checking, our children constantly challenge us to magic away their gripes as only parents can do. So you'd better be armed with an arsenal of pain-busting weapons – and perfect your brightest kiss-it-better bedside manner.

Trusters or cynics?

The first thing to do is to establish what variety of child you have: trusting believer or pragmatic cynic. Maxine has two children, Marnie, nine, and Freddy, three. "Freddy is a complete convert to the 'magic kiss'," she says. "As long as I give any little bump or pain the magic kiss, then he is away and playing again in seconds. Marnie, however, has always been far too cynical to think that that would work."

The trusters are simpler, obviously. My daughter Evie is a truster, in that she has always believed that some variety of cream plus a Winnie the Pooh plaster will fix anything.

Unfortunately she is also a complete wimp when it comes to a scrape or the tiniest amount of blood – she will sink into soft, inconsolable sobs for hours if the offending wound is left uncovered. The good news is that once covered up, the wound is forgotten and all is well again. Ahh, the times I have fashioned an impromptu bandage out of a wet wipe while out and about – works wonders, even if it does make her look like an extra from *Children's Hospital*.

Cynics take a little more effort than a plaster and a kiss. With these children, you have to be creative. Often, they will place their faith only in one particular remedy – a certain medicine, for example. "Marnie, at the age of about three, developed a bit of a thing for medicine," remembers Maxine. 'She started to ask for it for any little ache and bump. In the end I used to give her a little bit of fruit juice or water on a medicine spoon, which normally sent her away happy."

Many of your child's complaints will not present you with much of a challenge – your instinct as a parent will tell you whether a quick kiss or something more devious is in order. For more unusual or borderline gripes, having a good relationship with your local doctors' surgery is invaluable.

This can be cultivated to a sophisticated degree. "Treat the doctor's receptionist as a god," says Caroline, mother of Heather, three, and Murray, one. 'She has the key to your solutions and if you treat her well, she will repay you with whatever you need. If I need an appointment, I first listen for who is answering the phone so I can return thanks with her name. I have mentally stored information about her beforehand – is she going on her holidays, does she have grandchildren etc – so I can give her some chat. Then I normally start not with 'Can I have an appointment?' but with 'I wonder if you can help me ... I'm not sure what kind of appointment I need. I know it's not urgent, but I think she needs to be looked at, what do you think I should do?' This gives her ultimate power. It never fails to get me a quick appointment, even if there are none left."

Caroline admits that her doctor's receptionist now knows who she is without even referring to her surname. "The golden rule is not to cry," she adds. "They are hardened to it. This woman is more important than the doctor, and when I arrive for this 'urgent' appointment, I thank her in a gracious, 'I don't know what I would do if it weren't for people like you' kind of way."

For complaints which don't require such charm offensives or subterfuge, however, the following tips have been gathered.

Baby stuff

- A drop of breast milk up the nose for a tiny baby with a bad cold – it acts as a decongestant. "Breast milk is one of nature's miracles," says Annie, Evie's grandmother. "It's also great for cracked or sore nipples if you're breastfeeding – just dab some on after a feed."
- Blocks or thick books under one end of the cot to elevate the head end for a baby with a cold – this lets the mucus drain away better.

- For colic – various parents (mostly at their wits' end, and claiming only varying degrees of success) have suggested swaddling, massage, a drink of sugar water (sugar dissolved in tepid water), cranial osteopathy, and rolling a pram over a homemade 'rumble strip' on the floor (use towels or rugs, or the strip between a carpeted and tiled room).
- For nappy rash, again a wide variety of suggestions, including: cold wet tea bags on the rash, or a muslin soaked in cold camomile tea; egg white on the rash; olive oil on the rash; aiming a hairdryer on a cool setting at a freshly-washed rash, before applying cream; Metanium cream (potent yellow stuff available from chemists – I personally vouch for this one. It gets rid of anything in a day, but keep it away from clothes as it stains beyond belief).

Teething

- Cool, crunchy stuff like frozen strips of cucumber or carrot.
- Cool, soft stuff like fromage frais, yoghurt, ice cream and rice pudding.
- Ice cubes in a bottle or lidded cup of diluted juice.
- Ice pops or lollies to suck on.

Coughs and colds

- A few drops of an essential oil such as lavender or eucalyptus oil, or of Olbas oil, on a damp flannel on the radiator, or on a small hanky near the pillow for stuffed-up noses and coughs. But be careful – essential oils, if drunk from the bottle, can kill a child. Lock the oils away.

- An extra pillow case, or a Moses basket sheet, over the pillow of a child with a bad cold – you can whip it off when it gets snotty, and replace, rather than washing the whole bed set.
- A dab of Vaseline around the nostrils and under the nose for a toddler with a cold who wipes roughly and ends up with a red nose – this has always worked for Evie, who feels very special when she gets her special 'nose stuff'. Alternatively, a little baby oil on a hanky to make it less abrasive.
- Baby wipes rather than tissues for noses – they don't 'shed'.
- Calpol in the little sachets in your bag at all times. "And teach your child to suck it straight out of the packet," advises Anji, mother of Callum, three. "You're not hunting around for a spoon, which then dribbles all down them, and there's no sticky spoon to take home with you."
- Administer disgusting-tasting antibiotics by adding to a cup of juice rather than giving straight.
- A hot water bottle in a furry case or wrapped securely in a thick towel, for a child with an earache to lay their head against.

Bumps, bruises and general maladies

- Dark-coloured flannels for wimps like Evie to deal with bleeding knees – it disguises the blood.
- Skin creams for heat rash or for eczema kept in the fridge to give extra cool relief in hot weather. "This really helps in summer," says Rob, father of Chloe, four.
- Baby oil on a cotton wool pad to wipe over stubborn plasters and make them easy to remove.
- For head lice, tea tree oil, or an 'electric' nit comb available from chemists – plus a reminder that this happens to all children, however clean their hair may be.
- The cooperation of your child's favourite soft toys or dolls. "We often involve Bear with us in the cleaning of wounds or rubbing things better," says Caroline. "Making the toy talk also works a treat, and is a good distraction."
- On this line, buy some small red stickers from a stationer if your child has chicken pox, and make teddy poorly too. Your child can then help advise teddy not to scratch his spots.
- Another chicken pox tip is giving your child a cotton bud or small paint brush so they can dab their own spots with calamine lotion. Or dilute a bit of lotion and put it in a small clean spray bottle for easy coverage.
- Chicken pox parties. Think gatherings for your isolated child with other children who have *already* had it – you

can decorate their room with spotty decorations, and bake spotty cakes. But beware suggesting getting together with children who have not had the illness – this can be a popular suggestion with some parents who would like to get it over and done with, but can be met with scepticism by health professionals. One friend of mine rang NHS Direct, with all good intentions and a responsible attitude, to ask whether it might be a good idea to take her little girl to the house of a friend whose child had chicken pox. The person on the other end was aghast, demanded to know whether my friend had had any other thoughts of 'harming' her child, and left my friend tearfully feeling like the worst mother in the world.

A word on vaccinations: this is a highly personal issue. The only thing I would say is – don't be an ostrich. Sticking your head in the sand and doing nothing because you're not sure what to do is the worst option, for your child and for society in general.

My tip here would be to inform yourself. Ask health professionals, ask other parents, ask your own parents, read articles. And when you feel that you have done that as thoroughly as possible, make a decision based on what you feel in your own heart is right for that particular child.

Don't judge other parents for their decisions. But equally, don't make your decision based on pressure from friends, family, your GP or the government. The buck stops with you – so do what you think is best. If this involves opting for a combined vaccination, do it knowing you have taken the best advice possible. If this involves taking another route, be prepared to defend your views. But don't do nothing – sooner or later, it will catch up with you.

Lastly, the most effective tip I have heard from anyone regarding general bumps, and which I use myself, is: keep a poker face. By this, I mean not gasping out dramatically or rushing over with flamboyant gestures of comfort when your child falls over or traps a finger. They take their cue from you – if you think it's bad, then they feel they probably should think so too, and so will roar obligingly. Often, if judiciously ignored, a perceived injury will be summarily overlooked by the wounded party – and many of the above tips will be rendered unnecessary for your brave soldier.

CHAPTER 4

Travel

Planes, trains and automobiles without the fuss

It doesn't matter whether you're heading for Nanny's house or New Zealand, that inevitable cry of "Are we there yet?" seems to start as soon as you've left your front drive. From as early as two years old, children seemed programmed to utter it – in the same way they appear genetically destined to need a wee five minutes after you've just left a service station. Before the age of two, the same sentiment is there – it's just expressed as a howl of bored despair instead.

And the first forays out of the house with a new baby can be truly terrifying. "Scary times," says Jo, mother of Archie, four, and Charlotte, two. "Have you put the seat in correctly? What if they poo or are sick? What if they don't stop crying? Do I know enough songs to keep them entertained? Do I choose kids' CDs that I can't stand, or get them into my favourite music? At least then if it all gets too much I can just turn up the volume so I can't hear the crying …"

Transporting a child or, even worse, twins or a whole tribe of children is enough to test the calmest of parents. But unless you want to live like a hermit until your children reach adulthood, travel of some description is a must. And this, thankfully, is an area where a few practical preparations can make all the difference.

Essentials

Firstly, the car. You need to have a two-pronged strategy here – preparation and distraction. Preparation involves stocking up your car with certain essentials:

- A coat, woolly hat or sunhat, sun cream, a change of clothes including extra pants/knickers, and wellies.
- An old towel, a roll of kitchen paper, carrier bags.
- A small pack of emergency rations – think non-perishable items such as small packets of raisins, cereal bars, juice cartons.
- Proper food and drink supplies for longer journeys. "Allow more than enough – you never know when you'll be stuck in a jam," says Jo. "And remember both directions."
- Caroline, mother of Heather, three, and baby Murray, agrees. "Take your own stuff so you don't have to go into the shops full of chocolate, and can avoid the 'I want' tantrum," she says.
- A white sheet to cover up burning back seats in hot weather.
- A bag of small toys.
- Wipes, wipes and more wipes.

top tips

Other more imaginative tips include:

- A toddler cup filled with ice for hot days. “It stays nice and cold, and we found Emily can’t sprinkle it all over the seats,” says Richard, whose daughter is two.
- A waterproof bag such as a child’s swimming bag or just a sturdy plastic bag as a receptacle for all things dirty and smelly that have to be washed – eg clothing, or ‘real’ nappies.
- Talcum powder. “It’s brilliant for getting sand off feet after the beach,” says Dan, father of Ned, two. “It also makes clammy legs and feet comfortable for the journey home.”

Time busters for cars

Once you are fully prepared with essentials, you need to raise the stakes and think distraction. Anything you do before the journey will buy you peaceful travelling minutes once you set off.

“Give them plenty of things to keep them occupied,” says Andrew, father of Eleanor, four. “Be prepared to work hard to entertain them. Make them excited about where they are going. And, as far as possible, don’t take on too much – try not to drive all day because you want to get it over with.”

Different things appeal to different children. “Archie had an ‘over the car seat’ toy with dangly things,” says Jo. “Charlotte didn’t ‘get it’ at all. Take plenty of toys, and if you have a 'thrower', keep enough to hand in the front that you can keep passing new ones across. If only we had Mister Tickle arms …"

Some good time-passing tips are:

- Books, games and drawing stuff. Try a lap tray – or maybe one of those TV dinner trays with a cushion underneath – for them to lean on.
- A bag of small treats or toys, wrapped up (this is essential – unwrapping takes up time.) Give out one toy every half-an-hour. A variation on this is Pass the Parcel.
- A magnetic drawing board, or electronic computer-style game.
- Sunshades for the windows which can be drawn on with washable pens.
- 'Spotting' games with small prizes. Who will be the first to spot a black and white cow/blue van/traffic light? Ben, father of Joe, nine, Abigail, six, and Lara, four, who remembers "countless painful experiences from many years of long journeys to deepest darkest France and to North Yorkshire", agrees. "Games are crucial. We have an ongoing challenge, like a team version of I Spy, where we split the car into two teams with one adult on each, and you get points for spotting things – five points for a yellow car, 10 for a car with a bike on the back, 50 for a ginger vicar on a motorbike carrying a chicken, that kind of thing. You can keep it going for hours."

- A 'designer' version of this can include a sheet, maybe laminated if you're so inclined, with pictures of road signs, logos, landmarks etc on for them to spot. "Archie now likes to know what all the road signs are," says Jo.
- But some mothers – especially those of boys – warn that anything too competitive can be a bad idea, particularly if you have more than one boy in the back seat. "Better to get them to team up and work towards a collective target, or compete against you," says Roni, mother of Jack, now 10, Ned, eight, and Hal, five.
- Favourite cuddly toys. "Especially the ones required for sleeping," says Jo.
- "A variety of CDs because they'll ask for the same one to be played again and again," she adds. "We take turns between their music and our music."
- Ben agrees. "Audio books are great too. When Joe was about five, and proving a bit of a challenge on long trips, we borrowed the audio book of the first Harry Potter. We didn't hear a peep out of him for eight hours. And all three love music, so we let them take turns to request songs – it teaches them to be patient and wait their turn … supposedly."
- And finally, says Jo, "The patience of a saint to answer all the questions."

If all this fails, says Caroline, go at night. "There's less traffic congestion, and the children sleep so it's far easier to concentrate," she says.

Also – a note on twins. This is such a challenge that Jane, mother of Ethan and Hannah, two, tries to walk whenever she can. "Much easier than getting them both in and out of car seats and getting the monstrosity of a buggy in and out of the boot – oh, the effort!" she says. "From the age of two going in the car gets easier though – I open one door and they both climb through the same door and into their car seats where I can strap them in. This is also good if you're parked on a busy road as they can both get in on the footpath side."

Georgia, mother of twins Holly and Callum, one, also suggests buying, if possible, a car with sliding doors – great even for one child, and a boon with twins. "With one baby, you can manoeuvre the car to allow more room on one side to get the baby seat out," she says. "With twins, you need to get a seat out both sides. Sliding doors mean you can get the babies out in any car park. Also, add 15 minutes to any journey time for twins – an extra seven or eight minutes each end for getting them in or out."

Flying high

Those who graduate with honours from the car travel class can brace themselves for the next big challenge: planes, trains, or any other kind of long–haul travel which involves you having to physically carry any distractions you might choose to bring along.

This is where imagination really comes into play. You have no boot to store toys, no receptacles to stash sticky/sicky/horrid stuff, and above all, no choice in exactly when you stop, go, take a break or just give up and head home.

On the plus side, for many children airports, ferry terminals and the like are fascinating and exciting places, and you might find yours will be carried along on a wave of wide-eyed wonder through much of the journey. So don't despair – just prepare.

I have to confess at this point that I was a terrible coward when it came to holiday travel with Evie [*for more on holiday destinations and inspiration, see the Holidays chapter*]. I am something of a control freak, and therefore felt compelled to plan every last detail of the trip beforehand with an eye for detail that left travel agents and gîte owners quivering in shock.

"But is the balcony enclosed?" I would ask. "Could a two year old squeeze through the gap? Does our door back onto the pool? Are there handrails on the stairs? Does the lake have a fence round it?"

The first time Evie went on a plane she was nearly two, and it was only as far as Majorca. I was petrified – you would have thought we were on an expedition to Bolivia. She could have travelled in my seat, but I insisted on buying one for her to sit in between me and her father. I was convinced I wouldn't be able to cope with a marauding toddler for three hours and no seat. She would cry, struggle, accost the pilot, I thought.

As it was, she loved the whole thing. Yes, the seat came in handy (under-twos have to sit on your lap for take-off and landing, but during the flight the pull-down tray alone kept her amused for over an hour). But to be honest, she probably would have done fine without it. She loved the flight stewards, she loved the airport, she loved the taxi which didn't have a child seat (gasp), she loved the pool which was, in fact, right outside our door, and she cheerfully stayed up until mid-evening every night while we ate despite the fact I had been convinced she would wilt without her regular 7pm bedtime.

And when our return flight was delayed until 2am, she delighted in careering around Palma airport's marble floors, seemingly on booster-charge, until obligingly falling asleep in my arms about 10 minutes from Stansted airport with a beatific smile on her face.

I am a worrier. And most of it was needless worry. Children are actually very resilient.

Caroline, a veteran Scotland-to-Stansted flier, believes a healthy cynicism is essential. "Never believe what the airline or ground staff tell you," she says. "I say I'm travelling on my own, so can I have my buggy at the gate please? They say no problem. But when I get there, I'm told I have to go to baggage reclaim. I reply that they'll need to help me to get there, and just hand them the baby/toddler/bag – they can't say anything."

She adds: "Pay the money to get help. You only pay £5 with the budget airlines to pre-board, and can also pay to get help in the airport. Go to the disabled help desk."

top tips

Best airport tips are:

- The cheapest, lightest buggy you can find. Take it instead of your usual all-singing heavy one. They don't need rain guards/hoods and so on in warm weather, and if it gets battered in the hold, it won't break the bank.
- A packet of balloons. Small, light, and a godsend for entertaining little people if delays occur.
- ID wristbands – or a phone number written on an arm in biro, at a push – for toddlers who might wander off in airports (or on the beach when you get there).
- A blow-up lilo. "We took one to Spain, and when we got delayed for hours at night at the airport, I blew it up for Jack to nap on," says Mark, father of Jack, two. "He thought it was a giggle, which improved his mood, and he also managed to sleep on it too, with his blanky and teddy."
- A pillow from home, and cuddly toys, for settling on long-haul flights. 'Smells make all the difference to them settling," says Anji. "I also take Callum's monitor which has a nightlight on it for when I get there, so I can sit outside on the patio while he sleeps."
- Drumstick lollipops for toddlers. "It helps pop ears, keeps them quiet and takes at least five minutes to eat." says Caroline.
- Sick bags. "They can be used to draw on, put money in as a pretend purse, play sweet shops, use for origami..." she adds.

- A nappy or pull-up – even for toilet-trained children. "A few of my friends have been stuck on the runway for an hour and you aren't allowed to use the toilet," says Caroline. "Nappies are better than a child having to wet themselves."
- If your flight doesn't call families to board the plane first, go to the front of the queue anyway – people are usually very understanding, and it's easier to settle babies when the plane's not so full.
- Dress children in layers – the plane's air conditioning can be chilly.

Caron, a veteran flier with her son Tom, four, also suggests:

- Pre-arrange your seat allocation – preferably near the loos.
- Pre-order a child's meal for the flight – it's helpful if it's roughly child friendly rather than beef bourguignon.
- Check the airline's policy on taking on board a car seat – some will let your child use it strapped into the main seat.
- I give Tom a budget of £5–10 to buy goodies at the airport (choices carefully supervised). He puts them in his own small hand luggage bag. Avoid toys with too many easily lost pieces – Lego and Play Mobil are a nightmare when the pirate's hat/car wheel vanishes underneath the seat in front or rolls down the aisle.
- Brush up on word games. If you can see someone clearly, but they are out of earshot (really important) try a guessing game. See that lady in the pink jumper? Do you think

she's married? What job does she do? Does she have children? What sort of car does she drive? The results can be quite hysterical (for you, that is; the children are usually very earnest).

- Beware too many snacks with sugar and additives. On one journey, when Tom was two, we made it through the flight but by the time we disembarked in America and encountered an oh-so-serious gun-laden passport control officer, Tom, having eaten his way across the Atlantic, finally let rip. The officer loudly demanded: "Ma'am, can you keep your son under control?" as Tom swung gaily from the chain barrier shouting obscenities such as 'bum', 'poo' and 'stink' and I wished I hadn't supplied him with eight hours' worth of fizzy drinks and sweets.

- If all else fails on the flight, lock yourself and your child in the loo. At least you can't see the frowns on the faces of the other passengers.

And for twins, a certain resignation that the trip will be hellish is also necessary. "There's no easy way," laughs Jane, mother of Ethan and Hannah. "Under the age of two they don't pay for a seat but you and your husband have to have an infant on your lap the whole time – not easy to eat. You just have to have a mindset that you will not be put off doing what you want to do. We always take two single buggies abroad instead of our double one as footpaths in Europe tend to be narrow or cobbled, and doorways aren't designed for double buggies. It's a challenge at the airport though, because one parent has to push the baggage trolley and the other pushes two single buggies. We have to rope our elder third child

Emily into pushing a buggy. But it is wonderful and encouraging how many strangers will offer help too."

Train tricks

top tips

Train journeys can often be more fun for children, especially those brought up on Thomas the Tank Engine. Tips to smooth the way are:

- "Take loads of things to do that the kids don't know about," says Roni, who frequently travels by train with her sons Jack, Ned and Hal. "I also take a little drawstring bag with folded pieces of paper. Every 15 minutes or so, one of them draws out a piece of paper and everyone does what it says. It might be an activity or food, so it could say 'pens and paper' or 'trip to the buffet' or 'flapjack' or 'I Spy'."
- Travel as light as possible. Ditch bulky prams and go for a lightweight buggy with as many toys and distractions as possible squeezed into the basket underneath. Wear a rucksack (and give toddlers and pre-schoolers mini rucksacks) to free up your arms.
- When faced with flights of stairs on platforms when you have a buggy or pram to carry, try following signs for disabled travellers – usually the universal blue symbol of a person in a wheelchair. These often lead you to hidden lifts and ramps.
- Try travelling at night. "Sleeper cars are great with kids, says Mark. They love the bunks. It's more expensive, but worth it for a long trip.

- Do a trial run. Look for a tourist train, a sightseeing one or one on a heritage site, and take them for a ride on it, says Anji. You can get them used to what trains feel like, and talk about a few safety rules as well.
- Reserve a window seat. If you're going as a family or group, ask to reserve two sets of seats facing each other, so that you have at least two window seats for the children.

Plane and long-haul travel, incidentally, is the one area where small babies come into their own. Yes, they need special places to sleep, so perhaps invest in a travel cot. But, especially if you're breastfeeding, they are actually very portable. Slings mean you don't have to do buggies at airports, and breast milk, or formula, mean you don't have to worry if there will be fish fingers on the menu. They can't crawl off into the pool, they don't get bored with the sand, they sleep a lot, and they pretty much think that wherever you are is the best place to be. Make the most of it while you can.

CHAPTER 5

Clothes

Designer labels or supermarket specials? Tutus in public?

To prospective parents, clothing is probably the one area of impending parenthood which conjures up all of the excitement and none of the trepidation of what is to come.

Even parents with a tribe of young children still go gooey if a new one is on the way and they happen to pass the 'newborn' rail in the baby clothes department.

Every one of us probably has an idea in their mind's eye of what they see their son or daughter looking like at certain ages … first pink dress, tiny dungarees, a preppy jumper and shirt or a cool streetwise T–shirt, pigtails and bows, trainers or boots. And for the first couple of years of your child's life, you can pretty much indulge in that picture, and pander to your own tastes.

The trouble comes when your son decides he wants a buzz cut not a bowl cut, baggy jeans not cords. Or your daughter says no to frills and dresses, and wants mini crop–tops and denim instead.

And after that initial 'tiny clothes' thrill, it also dawns on you that:

- Clothes are expensive.
- Clothes shrink and go grey and get stained – despite being expensive.
- Your child will at some point have to dress themselves.
- Your child will refuse to wear certain things, and maybe even want to choose their own clothes in the shops.
- Your child will at some point insist on wearing a fancy-dress outfit in public, probably when your most glamorous, childless, work colleague is passing and you wish you were with a child that looked like a catalogue model rather than a Power Ranger with a penchant for fairy wings.

Practicalities

So, where to start? Firstly, I would advise you to do a limited bit of indulgence shopping. Go out and buy that impossibly impractical tiny frilly dress or cute pair of dungarees. Do it before your child is even born. This is the thrilling, exciting bit of expecting a baby, and don't let anyone make you feel guilty about it. Get the fix, hang it in the wardrobe, then – and only then – take a deep breath and get practical.

Some people will tell you to buy clothes only in unisex colours. This is a little difficult when you're yearning to go pink or blue and the prospect of another baby years down the line seems too remote to bother about.

"When buying for Archie, we bought plenty of unisex clothes in greens, yellows and reds but when you have a girl second, you do want to put them in pink when they're young," says Jo, mother of Archie, four, and Charlotte, two. "But things like wellies, raincoats and anything that will last a while we try to buy in unisex." Also, vests, sleep suits and basic bed linen such as sheets can be bought in white, with a few coloured touches like blue or pink dressing gowns and booties to liven things up.

Be hard-headed with quantities – you will inevitably get lots of new clothes bought for your baby by other people, as well as possibly hand-me-downs from an existing sibling or cousins and friends. You don't need to buy in bulk. "Don't buy too much," says Jo. "We have clothes that didn't get worn. Nothing wears out until they are crawling."

Caroline, mother of Heather, four, and Murray, one, adds: "Don't take the tags off new baby pressies until you see what you have got. We got lots of outfits which wouldn't be right for the season – shorts for December in Scotland – we weren't ungrateful, but you have to be practical."

And yes, clothes do get stained, but think bibs. Evie kept up a nice line in sicky burps for the first year of her life, so bibs were the fashion accessory we went for. "Bibs go with everything," agrees Jo. "Both of mine had to wear bibs – that's more than one at a time – for months, so get nice ones. And if you get the plastic-backed ones, wash them straight away or they go mouldy."

top tips

Other baby clothing tips include:

- Buy 0-3m sizes rather than newborn sizes – cuffs can be turned up, baggy feet do not matter, and newborn clothes only last about two weeks for most babies.
- Buy sleep suits without enclosed feet – they last longer.
- Adapt sleep suits for summer use by cutting off the legs to make shorties.
- Soak bibs in sterilising fluid to get rid of bad stains.
- Keep tiny baby clothes for your child to use as dolly clothes when they get a bit older.
- Co-ordinate. "There's no point buying something that goes with nothing else," says Jo.
- For babies who have learned to unzip their sleeping bags, turn the bags inside out – more fiddly for you to do up, but a real challenge for them to undo.
- All-in-one sleep suits or outfits must have poppers all the way up the leg to allow you to get to the nappy. And sleep suits with poppers up the back, rather than the front, may allow for cute designs on the chest but think about it – would you feel comfortable going to sleep on a row of metal studs?

Money matters

You will probably find that it's when your child hits older toddler age that you will be bought fewer clothes by family and friends. This coincides with your child needing more clothes because they are mobile and wearing them out faster, and with the clothes themselves costing more.

So this is when you have to get clever with money. These days, you're not just limited to the high street. There are many mail order companies that do fantastic children's clothing, and you also have the supermarket option, as well as, at the other end of the budgetary scale, designer wear.

But don't just think pounds – think quality. "Sale shopping for designer clothes is good," says Jo. "They do last longer. Buy at the supermarket if you know it will get trashed quickly or it can't be seen. The cheaper clothes tend to fade after one wash, shrink, go out of shape, or bobble. They're tempting – especially when they're in the only shop you have time to go to – but it's usually a false economy."

Caroline isn't sure. 'Supermarket clothes work for me the best as I'm not very good at getting the food stains out. Designer clothes often are different in sizing and the buttoning of the outfits in the wrong place – a newborn sleep suit that buttons up the back is a pain to do but also can't be very nice to lie on. I'm a sucker for the trendy slogan T–shirt though."

If you don't have older children to hand down clothes, why not get together with friends, or a mother and toddler group? "Our mums' group does a kind of 'clothes bank' between about 10 of us," says Anji, mother of Callum, three. "We store clothes in one of the mum's utility room, and we can go along and make deposits and withdrawals, just like with a toy bank."

top tips

Good money-saving tips:

- Use up odd socks by letting your children wear them in the house – or prevent misplacing them in the first place by using the little drawstring bags which come with washing powder tablets to contain them in the washing machine or tumble drier.
- If the legs are too short but the waist still fits, cut jeans into cut-offs for summer.
- Buy mittens and gloves in duplicate or more, so that if one goes missing you can still make up a pair instead of buying new ones.
- Buy easy-care clothes which can go in the tumble drier – otherwise that expensive dress will stay unworn in the wardrobe for weeks because you haven't had time to iron it.

Fashion victims

When your child becomes interested in their own clothes, they will probably begin to dress up, not only in fancy dress, but in whatever takes their fancy in their own wardrobe. This is the time to encourage them to start dressing and undressing themselves, in preparation for nursery and school (most will expect them to do so for PE).

"Archie never showed any interest in doing it himself," says Jo. "And because we're normally in a rush, we hadn't noticed we were still dressing him when he could/should have been doing it himself. We started at bedtime when there's more time. We took off the hard stuff and got him to do the rest and put dirty clothes in the washing basket (teach them this young). We taught buttons on his pyjamas, and where the label goes. Charlotte, on the other hand, already likes to 'do it herself'."

"Our problem isn't with getting dressed, it's a naked Heather we have a problem with," says Caroline. "She spends most of her days in her knickers or her leotard for dancing. I've started to make the house colder, which is having some effect."

Things that make it easier for young children to dress and undress themselves are:

- Tops with designs on the front, so they can tell which way is which.
- Teaching them to look for a label in the back, or marking the back with a laundry pen if there is no label.
- Teaching them to line up buttons and poppers from the bottom up – they find this much easier to do than from the top down.
- Bows or designs on girls' knickers – boys' pants are much easier because of the distinctive design at the front.
- A drawn picture, letter or sticker inside their shoes on the outside edge so they can recognise which goes on which foot.
- Dampening shoe laces before tying. "If you just squirt on a bit of water, they make a much tighter knot when they

> dry which doesn't come undone as easily," says Mandy, mother of Ben, four.

Once they've got the idea of independent dressing, they will probably start to take much more notice of what their friends are wearing – especially once they start pre-school. So do you let them pick out their own clothes?

"Last week at the shops Heather asked: 'Can I have a pair of high heels and a tattoo?'" laughs Caroline. "I nearly fell over with shock and said no. She said I'd ruined her life and stormed off. It later turned out she had meant 'tutu' …"

"My tip is to give them a choice – but a limited one," says Piers, father of Olivia, three. "I know Victoria (Olivia's mum) does this. Whether it's at home, or very occasionally if we're out clothes shopping, she won't say 'Which one do you want?' but 'Do you want to wear the jeans or the pink trousers?' or 'Will it be the red cardigan or the yellow one?' That way, Olivia feels like she's making a grown-up choice, and we feel like she's not going to leave the house looking like a rag doll."

If you haven't got time for discussions – a busy morning just before pre-school or nursery, for example – try choosing and laying out an outfit the night before.

Clothing choices for twins, especially identical ones, can be trickier. For times when you want to have your children recognised as individuals, it might be better to encourage them to dress differently. If they're in uniform, help teachers distinguish between them by using different coloured hair toggles for girls, perhaps, or watches, socks, shoes or wristbands for boys. You could also co-ordinate outfits rather than match them identically – the same outfit, for instance, but in a different colour.

And if your little one is dead-set on heading out of the front door in full Spiderman mode, or dressed in more plastic fairy bling than Barbie at a High School prom?

It all depends on the strength of your constitution. Some mothers make it a steadfast rule that all fancy dress comes off before exiting the house. Others feel that it's a battle not worth fighting – anything for a smiley face. And some think that if a child can't have a little sartorial fun when they're under five, there's something wrong with the world. "Archie has never asked," says Jo. "Charlotte, though, loves her pretty dresses which include fairy outfits. She looks cute – so why not?"

CHAPTER 6

Cleanliness

Hand washing and bathtime hints; tidy rooms and muck busters

It may dawn on you, during those first few weeks with a new baby, that once you are a parent your relationship with cleanliness may never be quite the same again.

What used to be a kind of 'silent habit' of personal and household cleaning and tidying will now require an ongoing battle plan, a grim determination and a good dose of craftiness to achieve. That old cliché about the Forth Bridge springs to mind.

The challenge is twofold: keeping your child clean (and helping them learn to do this themselves), and keeping everything they come into contact with clean.

Personal hygiene

Let's start with the first one. Actually, I think keeping the child itself clean is probably the easier of the two. After all, most dirt disasters can be tackled either with a handful of wipes or a bath. But what about encouraging your child to want to do it themselves?

Making bathtime fun is the obvious approach. If they think having a bath is an extension of play time, they're more likely to hit the suds. But sometimes a firm approach is also necessary. Caroline, mother of Heather, four, and Murray, one, says: "I tell Heather that if she wets the bed, she has to have a bath – she very quickly stopped wetting the bed to avoid the bath, which was a different problem solved."

Caroline used a children's hand wash "for initial potty training" but found the novelty soon wore off. "I'm trying to scare her into washing her hands by saying the germ creature in the TV bleach adverts will come and get her if she doesn't," she laughs.

Maxine, mother of Marnie, nine, and Freddy, three, also used scare tactics. "Marnie remembers washing her hands as a toddler to beat the germ monster," she says. "I think we managed to make him redundant in the end."

As for bath time, she says: "Forget expensive bath toys – Freddy in particular has ignored them all. Give him a couple of big plastic jugs from the kitchen and he'll stay in the bath for hours given half a chance. Getting him in the bath – especially if Marnie is already in there – isn't the problem, but I could do with tips on how to get him out."

top tips

Other top tips are:

- For reluctant hair washers, let them hold cotton wool balls over their eyes, or a flannel. "Or let them put on their swimming goggles – Ben thinks this is fantastic," says David, whose son Ben is four. "He even takes a snorkel in there too, sometimes."

- In cold weather, leave the shampoo bottle in the water for a few minutes before using, to warm the shampoo.
- Consider 'character' wash mitts to encourage washing. These can talk, give kisses, dive under the water etc. Evie has an Archie one from Balamory and an Australian one with a different outback creature on each finger. They have proved great bathtime friends.
- Stick pictures or glowing stars high on your bathroom wall or ceiling to encourage your child to tip back their head for hair rinsing.
- For babies who wriggle during nappy changes, try putting an interesting picture on the ceiling above their changing mat. Or give them something to hold, such as a child's plastic hand mirror. "We put a sticker on Milly's hand," says Jake. "She's so busy trying to get it off, she doesn't notice what's going on further down."
- Keep packets of wipes upside down to keep the moisture filtered through to the wipes nearest the opening – dry wipes make for grouchy children.
- For reluctant teeth brushers, make up a game. I used to pretend Evie's mouth was a house, and we'd make sure we cleaned the bedrooms, and the kitchen, and the living room.
- Buy two brushes, one for you to hold, and one for your child.

"Or try an electric toothbrush," says Anji. "Callum wasn't interested at all in brushing his teeth until he had a go with my electric brush. In the end I bought him one of his own."

- Let them clean their teeth in the bath. They can always rinse in the sink afterwards.
- Or sit them on your lap facing forward, and brush their teeth from behind – it's much easier than doing it facing them.
- And for muck that won't shift with a few bath bubbles, try baby oil or eye make-up remover (the oily sort) for getting rid of Biro and fun non-permanent tattoos/hand stamps on skin.

Stopping the muck spreading

If only cleaning everything else was so simple. The best approach seems to be to offset at least a little of the potential dirt-and-chaos factor in advance by setting up some kind of system to help your child keep their environment clean.

Let's not be too anal here – children are supposed to get a bit dirty. It's part of being a child. It's bad enough that these days few of us feel comfortable sending our children out for the day to play endlessly on their own in mucky streams or meadows or woods or even kick about on the street – if we then blitz them with bleached perfection when they are at home, we will turn out a generation of pernickety neat freaks with no immune systems.

However, a little order is usually required for the sanity of the rest of the family. So here goes.

Make some space for your child to do stuff – mucky stuff. Instead of worrying where the paint or Play-Doh is going, spread out a plastic tablecloth and let them dig in. Buy plastic aprons, put them in their oldest clothes and then chill out.

Their own rooms are less likely to get the 'let's cover the entire carpet so you can't see it any more' treatment if they have different areas for different things. Even tiny rooms could have an area for reading (if only the bed or a small chair), one for drawing, one for dolls or cars, one for games, and so on. And they're much more likely to help tidy up properly if they have specific places to put things. Evie has a nice line in see-through pink plastic boxes from a stationery superstore. "If you're really brave, you could try colour-coding," says David. "You use drawers or shelves in bright colours, then put corresponding stickers on the toys. I've seen this done in pre-school and it works, to an extent."

To encourage them to be organised:

- Put little bits and pieces in see-through boxes. They can see what's inside, and what goes where.
- Use open-sided boxes or cubes stacked along a wall for storing bricks, cars, dollies etc.
- Get them into the habit of helping tidy up before bed. Create games to see who can do it the fastest, or give a small bedtime prize for the cleanest room. If they learn they have to deal with their own mess, it might not grow to such drastic proportions.

Dirt busting

Of course, no matter how prepared you are, you will end up with clothes, carpets, sofas and walls bearing the marks of your little one's creative efforts or accidental messes.

So what happens when the gunk hits the fan? Don't panic. Enlist some help – even from your child, if no one else is handy. And, of course, reach for the wipes.

"Baby wipes are superb for getting stains out of carpets,"says Maxine. "One friend even got some paint off the carpet using them. I have used them for spilt moisturiser on carpet too."

They are also great for getting food stains off clothes when used straight away, and for getting mud off suede or nubuck shoes and boots. But when wipes don't cut it, try these:

- Use dilute lemon juice in hot water to lift nappy cream out of carpets with a scourer or nailbrush.
- Use hairspray to get crayon and pencil off walls. Wipe off gently and go over again with a damp cloth.
- To remove trodden-in Play-Doh, let it dry, then use a nail-brush or suede brush to lift, then vacuum up the small lumps.
- Ice cubes are apparently great for tackling chewing gum. "Peanut butter works too," says Liz, mother of Lily, two. "Especially in hair. You rub it in gently, and it lifts it out."
- Baking soda on baby sick gets rid of the mess and the smell. Leave to absorb, then vacuum.

- Furniture polish lifts stickers off surfaces. Leave for a few minutes then wipe off.
- A drop of washing-up liquid in powder paints makes them a lot easier to clean after the masterpiece has been created.
- Having a tiny entrance hall, I love this one: keep a dustpan and brush on the doorstep or near the front door to get the worst mud off buggy wheels in the winter.

Finally, remember that the only way your child will learn to help you keep their home clean (and stand any chance of not turning into a teenager who expects you to skivvy for them) is to get them involved at an early age.

Don't be a dragon – make it fun. Many children love it when you enlist their help – and not just girls. Boys will have fun with a broom or a feather duster too. If you've got one of those hand-held vacuum cleaners, so much the better. Brushes, dusters and wipes will often be enthusiastically received – and even if they don't actually clean very much, at least they will be occupied while you scurry round.

"Jackie and I sometimes clean the bathroom while Esme is in the bath," says Peter. "It means one of us can get something done while still making sure she is safe. I give her a wipe to 'clean' the tiles round the bath with, which she loves, while I do the rest – and then I do the bath itself quickly once she's out."

Keeping clean – whether it's babies, pre-schoolers, carpets or walls – can become something of a preoccupation for stressed parents. Just remember, as long as it's healthy enough for your child and acceptable enough for you, that's fine. Recent guidelines suggest that a bath three to five times a week is fine for a child – in fact, a bath every night may even exacerbate skin conditions in some children. And our parents and grandparents survived just fine without the latest armoury of anti-bacterial products on offer today.

Don't think clean. Think clean enough. That's all you and your children need right now, and all anyone else can expect.

CHAPTER 7

Potty training

How to take the plunge, and how to avoid puddles at home or out and about

Potty training is hideous. Let's be very clear about that. Helping a small person with an attention span that struggles with your average Balamory storyline to anticipate their own bodily functions while getting to grips with zips, buttons and elastic is never going to be a breeze.

Go into this with your eyes wide open and your carpets on red alert, and you will find it a whole lot easier. This is not the time for denial.

Some experts will advise you not to refer to this stage as potty training at all, but instead to call it potty learning. Your toddler is not a dog, they reason; they are acquiring a new skill, not receiving electric shocks for getting it wrong. This is an admirable stance; whether or not you will stick to it after you have just scraped poo off your fourth pair of Barbie knickers or Thomas pants in an hour is debatable. I prefer to call it war.

Call to arms

In order to remain calm when all about you is soggy or soiled, you will need to gather an arsenal of weapons. Potties, obviously – but lots of them. One for upstairs, one for downstairs, one for nanny's house, one for the car … a standard model costs only a few pounds, so invest in as many as you can. The reasoning behind this is that the nearer your child is to one, the more chance they have of hitting their mark. It also sets out your intentions clearly: the potties are here. You can run, but you can't hide.

Variation is another tool. Evie had a nice line in small pink potties which she was perfectly happy to play with, put on her head, use as a handy crisp dispenser and so on, but not to use as a receptacle for wees and poos. She wouldn't even sit on one with clothes on. When we took a special trip to buy a larger potty seat – a commode-style affair with a back and sides and a removable pot – she was, within hours, ensconced on the throne in front of the television with all the relish of a miniature Jim Royle.

Other weapons:

- Own roll of toilet paper (yes it does end up festooning your living room in the manner of a prison riot but it encourages a great sense of pride).
- Own plastic box of kiddies' toilet wipes (you may think these unnecessary or a sell-out, but they make them feel grown-up and, anyway, moist is the way to go when you're

trying to help wipe a bottom that's hovering precariously over your best rug).

- A protective sheet for under the potty (or, better, an old bath mat from the airing cupboard).
- Good carpet stain remover (or a quick conversion to hard floors).
- For the pet-friendly, apparently cat litter does wonders in absorbing accidents on carpets and getting rid of odour – just vacuum it away afterwards.
- Distraction (dollies or teddies to keep company, favourite DVD, tape of songs you can join in with – and you. Potties are far less daunting if you are sitting on the floor next to their occupant. How vulnerable would you feel if you had to do your business surrounded by towering furniture and an open expanse of draughty floor?)
- Optional extra: baby doll that wees. Some experts (mostly American, for some reason) swear by these. My daughter quickly grew rather ratty with her model's gleeful incontinence, frowning with suspicion at the rather startling hole in its rear end.

The battle plan

Once you have stocked up, you are ready to begin. I am in favour of a two-pronged strategy to start with: cold turkey combined with strong incentives (yes, I mean bribery).

Cold turkey means proper pants at all times other than when sleeping – at least, initially, in the home. "Buy the most highly decorated ones you can find – princess knickers, train pants – the more highly festooned with recognisable characters, the better." says Richard, father of two year old Emily. "Emily went on a special shopping trip with her mother to get hers." Buy at least 20 pairs. And shop for them together, then let them try them on for a couple of days before bathtime, or even over a nappy. Show them yours – let them see they have 'Big Girl's Knickers' or 'Big Boy's Pants' too.

If you have been using ordinary nappies, announce their departure as if it has been an act of God rather than anything to do with you. "Guess what – we haven't got any of your nappies any more. We can't go and buy them because the shop hasn't got any. What shall we do? Shall we try your knickers instead?"

Then stock up on pull-up style nappies, and call them 'Night–time Pants' or 'Bed Knickers'. These, you explain, are not real nappies like their old ones, but special knickers for when they're asleep only, or if you have to make a long trip out of the house to a place where there are no potties. The minute you return home or they wake up, off comes the pull-up and on go the ordinary knickers.

The reason cold turkey is best is that, if you dilly-dally about with the idea of proper underwear and only use it when it's convenient, not only will you confuse them, but you will string out the whole process. They need to feel that you are both working together to solve a problem that neither of you has any power over – the lack of nappies.

It's you and your child against the world – and that's hard to pull off if you chicken out just in case they wee on grandma. Again.

Incentives, then:

- Stickers work well. Most children's bookshops have story books about using a potty which come with a sticker chart in the back – but you can also make your own. A racing car track for boys, maybe, or a fairy path through the woods for girls, with a toy or trip when they reach the end.
- Hand stamps can also do the job – use face paints for easy removal. Children can then show these off: "I got four stamps today, Daddy."

If, however, your toddler (like mine) typically treats all new experiences with staunch resistance, you may have to play dirty. Yes – I mean edible treats. Sorry, but it works. When all else fails, you've just mopped up your seventh puddle of the morning and you are starting to consider taping your child's bottom to the pot, it works.

- Buy a large plastic box with a lid, announce that this is The Potty Treat Box, and stock it copiously. Use your judgement here – the idea is not to present them with their own corner sweetshop and a fast ticket to a gummy smile. Think small – little boxes of yoghurt-covered raisins, packets of dried fruit from the health shop, the odd lollipop. And stick to the rule – one treat for every wee or poo. A 'try' isn't good enough – they have to produce the goods.
- If you can't bring yourself to compromise their pearly

> whites, go for a 'surprise bag' of small – very small – gifts instead. Or be really imaginative. One mother I know made up a little song that she and her husband sang every time their daughter's bottom hit the potty – with a nice little add-on variation when a wee or a poo was produced.

At the potty stage, it's all about practice and reminders. Aim is less of a problem for girls than for boys, so give boys an incentive to get it right. "With boys it's all about aim," says Nic, mother of pre-schooler Liam, four. "A good trick is to put a ping-pong ball or similar-sized ball in the potty, and get them to aim the stream of wee at it." This can be made into a game, with rewards for a good shot. And according to Georgia, mother of Woody, four, a favourite pre-school trick once they progress to toilets is to fix a sticker to the back of the toilet bowl as a target.

A note on coping with twin training – it doesn't get much harder than this. Jane, mother of twins Ethan and Hannah, two, says that most advice is to potty train twins individually. She disagrees. "I found this impossible as they always want to copy what the other one is doing," she says. "If you can get through the first 48 hours of permanently tipping potty contents down the toilet and spraying anti-bacterial spray on everything in sight, it's actually a good thing to do them both at once. Having one watch and copy the other is really helpful if one child is particularly reluctant. Choccie buttons for Number Ones and two choccie buttons for Number Twos also helps."

Once you've made the transition from potty to toilet, getting to operate the flush works as a reward for some intrepid children – although it frightens others. Big toilets sometimes require a little extra imagination and lateral thinking. Here are some tips:

top tips

- One idea – not one for neat freaks – is to put flushable items such as confetti or coloured ice cubes in the toilet water – this not only provides admirable toddler amusement, but also target practice.
- Anji, mother of Callum, three, adds a twist: "Dye the toilet water with food colouring – it changes colour when the wee hits."
- Jon, father of Sam, two, suggests: "We put him on backwards. He could hold on better, and aim easier. After a while, he got more confident and started standing up for wees."

Once you find that your child is willing, but easily distracted, you might find a reminder is helpful for you both. A timer – set initially for every half-an-hour or so, and gradually increased as they get more reliable – will pre-empt most accidents and will eventually prove unnecessary as they beat the clock anyway.

Timing, incidentally, is a key sneaky tool in another sense: don't start too soon. It's all too easy to be cowed into potty training by judgmental grandparents who swear they had you out of nappies before you could walk, or by a boastful Supermummy whose precocious two year old happily takes herself off to the toilet "and even insists on washing her hands all by herself afterwards".

The fact is, children vary enormously in being ready to give up nappies. Many children are three or older before it's time. If, when you try, it is clear they have absolutely no idea when they are ready to wee, you're pushing too fast. So here's a tip: don't let on that the attempt failed. Just put the nappy back on ("Look! The shop got some more in"), say nothing and try again a few months later. You'll be saving yourself a lot of soggy floors, and your child a miserable time of feeling like a failure when it's simply a case of bad timing.

Be aware also that you can't turn back the clock, which you may well wish to do when it dawns on you that you no longer have the safety blanket of a nappy when you venture outside. It's scary, believe me. A simple trip to town requires knowledge of all handy loos and potty stops. Ask your friends with older children, for they will have already worked out all the craftiest and cleanest conveniences and have a mental network of them tattooed on their minds. When one friend told me about the loo hidden at the back of the children's department in our local bookshop I nearly wept with gratitude.

Cars, too, need forethought. An absorbent disposable changing mat laid double in the car seat provides reassurance. Always take a car bag with extra pants, wipe and a change of clothes in it. "If the worst happens, the hand dryers in the loos in public toilets and in motorway rest stops are powerful enough to do an emergency drying of a car seat cover," says Dan, father of Ned, two.

Night-time tactics

You will know when you have been promoted to the ranks of the smug 'almost there' toilet training brigade when you start worrying about night-time. "Dry in the day" is a phrase you will hear often, with the unsaid "… but not in bed" hanging grimly in the ether. My tip? Wait.

Some statistics show that as many as one in 10 six year olds still regularly wets the bed at night. This can run in families, and can be worse with boys than with girls. The accepted rule of thumb is that once you start getting dry nappies/pull-ups in the morning, you can give it a go.

Most parents seem to think that restricting liquids before bed and 'lifting' a half-asleep child onto the loo in the middle of the night simply do not work. My mother very practically advises me to make a kind of 'sheet sandwich' with a sheet, a waterproof layer and then another sheet on top so that if an accident does occur in the night, the top two can be taken away and a dry one is there waiting for you without the need for midnight airing cupboard rummaging.

I believe the best strategy is to hang on until, one day, your child is simply physically and mentally ready – and they let you know. Until then, save yourself the stress. Who sees their tell-tale padded bottoms in bed anyway?

Whatever stage you're at though – first tinkles or finishing touches – there comes a time when you're convinced it's now or never, you have polished your weaponry of tricks, shortcuts and methods of pure bribery, and you have to take a deep breath, stand back – and grit your teeth.

There *will* be accidents – sometimes many, many of them. These must be treated with a kind of brisk insouciance in the manner of a kindly postmistress: "Oh dear, well, never mind, let's just clear that up for you and then you can try to get there in time next time. Remember, when you've got pants on, you have to tell mummy if you can feel a wee-wee in your bottom …" (It helps to try to convey to a child that you get a 'feeling in your bottom' when you need to do a wee – initially, they simply don't realise when one is coming and it is as much of a surprise to them as to you when it does.)

If, at the end of a long day, your postmistress façade is slipping and you fear you may well turn into a kind of barbaric dog trainer and rub their nose in it instead, walk away. Take a deep breath, and walk away. It's only wee. It's not even red wine. Remember – this is war.

Don't let your mask slip. You will not be beaten by wet knickers. Go into the kitchen, find something nice in the fridge to distract yourself, then return with a smile – a big one. Teeth showing. Teeth, I said, not fangs.

CHAPTER 8

Manners

Ps and Qs, pre-school etiquette, and the art of defusing the toddler tantrum

Manners mean different things to different people. Some of us might expect our children to behave like a miniature Jane Austen character with beautifully polished social skills by the age of three. Others might consider themselves lucky if their child manages a trip to the supermarket without leaving behind a trail of sniffy shoppers with aghast expressions on their faces.

So the first thing to do when teaching manners to your child is: establish your own standards. What exactly do you expect? Are you consistent? What is important to you, your wider family, and your social circle – and do you care enough about this to enforce it?

Personally, for instance, I don't feel it necessary that Evie address every adult she meets by their title and surname – a polite first name with a good dose of pleases and thankyous will do. I also hate that old-fashioned custom of making children address unrelated adults as Auntie and Uncle. But I do insist that she helps write her own thank you notes, that she sits at the table until she is given permission to get down, and that she shares her toys. We're still working on that last one.

Most people would probably say their expectations of good manners fall into a few broad categories:

- Respect – for themselves, you, other adults and their peers.
- Tolerance and patience – the ability to wait, not to interrupt, to accept different people and ways of doing things.
- Fair play – learning how to share and take turns.
- Social graces – table manners, phone etiquette.
- Controlled behaviour – no tantrums.

Some children get the hang of one or more of these early on. "Heather is a strange one, as her manners are generally good but slightly eccentric," says Caroline, whose daughter is four. "She asked her little pal if he would like to 'join her for tea', which raised a few smiles. But her behaviour after sugar is awful."

A case in point – no child is perfect. That friend of your son or daughter who comes to tea and appears to have perfect table manners, putting your child to shame, quite probably goes home to stage diabolical tantrums about going to bed, or having a bath. A sweetly polite telephone message taker may have no idea how to share his favourite toy without a United Nations-scale peacemaking effort by any adults in the vicinity.

So, right from the start, take a deep breath and forget perfection. Sometimes your child will be polite, and sometimes they'll forget. But they'll be no worse than anybody else's child – and with a little sneaky encouragement, a whole lot better.

Next, remember that you can't start encouraging manners too early. Even tiny toddlers can learn to say thank-you. One of the best ways to teach them to say thank-you is when you hand them anything – a cup or toy for example. Don't let go until they say it. They quickly cotton on to why you're not handing it over.

Most of the best tips on manners are the sort that should just become seamlessly absorbed into your daily life. Suddenly embarking on a regime to install good manners when a child is five will be an uphill task and lead to a confused and bombarded child. In fact, most experts agree that you should concentrate on one 'social skill' at a time – table manners, let's say, or phone manners – and focus on just that for around a month before moving on to something else.

Etiquette and social stuff

Think 'show, don't tell'. Sneak in some bits and pieces that make good manners fun – a special pink phone pad by the phone for messages, maybe, or Thomas the Tank Engine cutlery. Smart bits and bobs like this will engage your child – and avoid you coming across like a starchy Victorian governess.

top tips

The 'practical' skills are often the easiest to teach. Best tips for good table manners, for example, include:

- Role play at 'tea parties', with 'polite' teddies and dolls gaining praise, and 'rude' ones being gently corrected. Sneaky parents will make sure there's always a 'rude' one. "Esme loves this," says Peter, whose daughter is three. "She gets a real kick out of being the one who knows how to do it right – and teaching it to her 'babies'."
- Sitting down as often as possible as a family round the dinner table and using cutlery rather than finger food. Make a game of it: "How many peas can you get on your fork?"
- Holding a 'special night' once a week. "Friday nights for us are 'restaurant night'," says Paul, mother of Mabel, three, Arthur, five, and Joshua, eight. "Marianne helps the children to set the table with a cloth and nice glasses, light a candle, and the children dress up in nice clothes – or sometimes fairy dresses for Mabel. Each week they take it in turns to choose the kind of food we eat, and help to prepare it. I get home from work an hour early on a Friday, so then we can all sit together and make sure we use our best table manners. We've been doing this since Arthur was little, and Mabel joined in even when she was in her highchair."

  Likewise, telephone manners can be fun to learn. Top telephone tips are:

- If you need to be able to take a call without interruptions, plan ahead. Keep toys or drawing stuff near the phone to distract your child.

- "We have a special signal that lets Olivia know if it's an important, no-interruptions call," says Piers, whose daughter is three. "If I, or Victoria, hold our hands up in a kind of 'time out' signal, she tries to be quiet. She has learned to respect that – most of the time."

- If it's a more casual chat that you can end when you want to, try using an hourglass-style sand timer to time your call so that your child knows when it will end.

- As they get older, encourage them to take messages by leaving a pen and paper by the phone. Some message pads have prompts for who called, the time they called, a return number and so on.

- Teach your child that, while it's important to be honest, callers don't always need to know everything – the fact that you are on the toilet, for instance. A simple "Can Mummy call you back?" will do.

- If it's important for a child to learn how to take messages properly, hold practice sessions. "I used to call our landline from my mobile while I was there in the same room, so that Ben could pick up the landline and practise what to say," says David, whose son is now four. "We started that last year and now he has a lovely telephone manner and even my work colleagues have commented on it."

When it comes to general respectfulness, tolerance and a sharing, caring attitude, this can be harder to explain to a small toddler, but should start early nevertheless. If you keep up the standard, the success rate when they get it right will gradually start to rise as they get older.

top tips

Good tips for encouraging thoughtfulness are:

- To get even small children to help send thank-you notes, get them to sit with you while you write, tell you something about the toy which you can transcribe, and adorn the card with a scribble, kisses, or maybe an initial or a scrawled name.
- Use a sand timer for siblings or friends learning to share toys.
- Use an empty jar as a rewards capsule. Every time they earn a reward through good behaviour or a display of good manners, put in something – a pebble, a marble, a piece of dry pasta, a cotton wool ball. At the end of the week, count the contents and exchange them for pocket money (5p per piece, for instance) or a treat, outing or favourite film. "We did this for Ben," says David. "We used marbles. He always exchanged them for either a trip to the swings or, if he thought he could get away with it, a chocolate egg when we did the supermarket shop."
- Teach children that actions have consequences. If they are rude, they have to say sorry. If they have a fit of temper and break something, get them involved in fixing it. If they have been mean to a friend, ask them to think of ways they could

do something nice for that person – paint them a picture, buy them a small gift.

Tantrum troubles

Experts will tell you that tantrums are common in two and three year olds and that they are a 'constructive' part of normal childhood development. Try reminding yourself of that when your darling is turning purple in the tinned goods aisle.

There aren't many children who don't turn on the tantrums at some point. But there are a few things you can do to avoid too many of them. And a few tips for managing them when they do occur.

The best avoidance advice I ever heard was this: children are far more likely to have tantrums if they are tired, hungry, uncomfortable or bored. So, where possible, avoid doing major tasks like an hour-long supermarket shop under the above conditions.

top tips

Good tips are:

- Go prepared. Take books, toys and finger snacks to get round the supermarket/shop/town centre. If you give food, make it as un-sugary as possible and as time-consuming to eat as you can.
- Go after a nap, and with a clean nappy or after a recent toilet trip.

- Give them a shopping list and ask them to 'spot' things you need. "We sometimes stuck labels, like baked bean labels or coffee labels, onto a sheet of paper for Esme to spot," says Peter. "It was worth the five minutes' preparation for an hour of easy shopping."
- If they keep asking for things, see it from their point of view – you have all the choosing power, and they have none. So when they ask, say "Let's write it down." Often this is enough to quell the tears. But you can also choose a couple of small items off the list at the end so that some of their choices were listened to.

If, despite all your preparation, the worst still happens, remember that all those people looking smugly aghast were children once too. Relax – if you tense up, your child will sense it and step up the decibel level even further. Negative attention is better than no attention in their book.

At this point, you could get on the floor with your child and attempt to 'out-tantrum' them and shame them into submission in the style of a well-known television advert, but few of us have got the stomach for this. If not, some other tantrum busters are:

- A simply tired and tearful child may respond to a cuddle. A more defiant one will need a talking to – but a low, authoritative voice is better than a despairing yell. It will make the child strain to listen to you, and will make you feel less like a screeching fishwife.
- Distraction often works if you catch a building tantrum

early enough. "I've been diverting a lot recently," says Caroline. "I'll say to Heather 'Come on, we're going to nursery' and she'll say 'No I'm not,' so I'll reply 'What's that smell? Is it your shoes? Oh, we can't go to nursery with shoes smelling that bad, you're right.' At this point, Heather replies defiantly that she wants to go to nursery, and the crisis is averted for a few hours."

- Other distractions might include breaking out in a silly song, or doing a dance (depending on your location and fortitude). My husband has a lovely line in manic dancing which has always stopped a mutinous Evie in her tracks.

- You might consider calling the tantrum behaviour by a special name – 'the nasties', for instance, or 'the stormies'. You can talk to your child in advance about how to recognise when 'the stormies' are coming, and how to beat them. This puts you and your child on the same side, and gives them a sense of control over their behaviour. It can sometimes even divert a potential display of anger into a fit of the giggles.

- A word of advice from Evie's grandmother Christine. "When you're punishing bad behaviour, never threaten anything you're not prepared to carry out – or promise something you can't give. Your word will mean nothing to them if you consistently do this." She's right – so don't say that big trip to the seaside is off if you are desperate to go. Choose a threat that you really can and will carry out, and one which doesn't make your day go to pot as well.

Role models

At the end of the day, the best tip of all is: be a good example. Even if it kills you. Bite your tongue, don't shout at other motorists, and don't say nasty things about your own acquaintances/mother-in-law/neighbour while your child is within earshot.

"Unfortunately, it's no good having one rule for children and another one for the adults," says Annie, Evie's other grandmother. "It sends them a mixed message. They learn from you about treating people properly, and about what is acceptable and what isn't."

One thing – it is difficult, at an age when you are trying to teach children about honesty and truthfulness, to explain that sometimes it isn't kind to say something which is true but hurtful. We've all cringed when our darling child has raised some gauche but accurate query along the lines of "Why is that lady's bottom so big?" or "What is that awful smell?", only to wail defensively (and loudly) "But it's true Mummy!" as you hurry them away apologetically.

"Ask them if they would be upset if their best friend said it to them," says Annie. "Explain that if it would make them sad, it's best not to say it to someone else, even if it is true."

And finally, remember that most children actually want to be nice. Honest! They *want* to impress you. It's just that social niceties have to be taught, and tantrums are a good way, if you're two, of finding out where nice ends and nasty begins.

"Children love to gain your approval," says Annie. "You just have to teach them how to do that. Children who have awful manners are either confused, have never been told how to do it, or don't know the boundaries and are trying to find them."

So set some boundaries – make sure you stick to them too – and hopefully, your child will follow suit. If not, get out that rewards jar – a little incentive can work wonders when it comes to Ps and Qs.

CHAPTER 9

Boy business and girl power

From war games to fairy outfits – do you give in to the stereotypes?

It's an issue parents have been preoccupied with going back many generations: what, exactly, are little boys and little girls made of? Are they intrinsically different – or do we make them that way? And if we treat them the same and give them the same toys to play with, will it have any effect on our fairy princesses, cowboys and tomboys at all?

However admirably we go into the parenthood game with high ideals about keeping an open mind, we all – *all* – of us inevitably bring some baggage to the matter of gender roles. Every day, we send out messages to our children about our own attitudes to their gender, and what that means in terms of myriad things including toys, outside play, rough and tumble, tears, hugs, clothes and toughness.

Same difference?

Some of us try the 'new age' approach. We dress our girls in primary colours, let our boys experiment with jewellery and fairy dresses, and make sure we dish out the dollies and the toy cars in equal measure. We avoid using those oh-so-easy labels – "She's a tomboy", "He's a sissy", "She's a bit shy", "He's such a little monster" – and we make sure both our boys and our girls get time tumbling around in the garden or cuddled up quietly with us on the sofa.

Others of us opt out of all of that. We actively encourage our boys to be 'little men' in their cute boots and dungarees, chuckling when they sit next to daddy on the sofa, all 'mini-me' with their legs akimbo, intently watching the football. We dress our girls in the flounciest of pink outfits – after all, they stay young for such a short time these days – and we smile tearfully when they coo softly to their dollies or pretend to do the ironing. And if, God forbid, daddy catches his little boy sidling up to that ironing board or cradling that dolly … it's off to the garden for an emergency boisterous kick about. (I'm convinced I've even caught my husband looking slightly uncomfortable if our baby boy Charlie spends too much time in Evie's very pink bedroom – in case Charlie somehow might 'catch' a dose of 'girlie'.)

But the thing is, on talking to lots of real parents, it doesn't matter how overtly we influence our children one way or the other – because they seem to go their own way whatever.

How many times have you seen a small boy from a household where toy guns have been banned race around shouting "Bang bang you're dead" with a banana, a stick, or, if push comes to shove, his finger? Or a girl who, with no dolls to hand, will attempt to wrap up a pet cat or a teddy or one of your best ornaments and push it around lovingly in a pram?

So, whether you go for traditional or 'new age', you need to get sneaky if you want a well-rounded child rather than a shrinking violet or a mini-commando.

"I had all these ideas about wanting my daughter to grow up into a strong, confident woman who could do anything, could compete with any of the boys," says Victoria, mother of Olivia, three. "I still want her to be like that – but I also realise that, right now, she wants to be a princess most of the time. If I took that away from her, I'd be taking away part of her self-expression. So princess she is – but I'll often suggest that she is the one rescuing the prince or fighting the dragon, rather than sitting in the ivory tower waiting for her knight in shining armour."

Equally, boys don't always do what you expect them to do. All geared up to combat an overdose of testosterone-fuelled aggression in their son Ben, four, parents Mandy and David were surprised when instead he showed a preference for dressing up and playing with his female peers. "I thought David would be freaked out at first," says Mandy, "but David tries hard to let Ben be himself – and in return, Ben humours his dad and still joins in some boy stuff with him, like football and bikes. Although I do notice that on days when David gets Ben up and dressed, Ben inevitably ends up with his manliest, most rugged outfits on."

According to studies, a baby starts to behave in a gender-stereotyped way before the age of one. One study even showed that monkeys display gender preferences – the baby monkeys were given various toys, and – you guessed it – the young males preferred the balls and cars, the females preferred dolls and a pot. They played equally with neutral toys such as a picture book and a stuffed dog.*

So, if the hormones kick in that early, is there any point in worrying about the influences of environment and home life? Probably not. Just accept that boys and girls will be different – but let them stretch their 'range'a bit. Let them have a variety of toys – dolls, homey stuff and things that encourage nurturing, *and* cars, trucks and action figures that lead to adventurous play – whether they're a boy or a girl. It won't compromise their femininity or masculinity, honest!

Boys, toys and noise

Best tips I've had for boys are:

- Try to avoid negative labels – are you describing your son as 'rebellious' for behaviour which, if you had seen it in your daughter, would be called 'spirited'? Children try to live up to those labels, so if it's a negative one, that's what you might end up with.
- If your son is a sensitive soul, teach him some coping strategies for when he's at school or in a place where other things are expected of him. Perhaps he's not at ease play-

*Gerianne Alexander and Melissa Hines, 2002. *Sex Differences in Response to Children's Toys in Nonhuman Primates.* Evolution and Human Behaviour, 23, 467–479.

ing football with his male peers – but maybe he's the best one at telling jokes, or collecting, or acting, or diverting teasing with a smart reply.

- Is your son a mini tornado at home? Get physical. "We got Josh a little 'chinning bar' which fitted across the door to his room with suction cups," says Paul, whose son is eight. "If he gets too rowdy, we charge upstairs and count him through ten chin-ups – he loves it, and it kind of defuses a lot of tension or aggression. You can start the bar really low and move it up as they grow."
- More than one boy in a household can be an extra challenge. Sneaky parents get rid of excess energy by making them think they're having fun. Remember, men have evolved from creatures made to be outdoors – so get them outside in the garden, or on the beach or in the woods if you can. Give them space and tools – a rake to rake up leaves, a trowel to dig in the mud. Boys cooped up inside together in front of the TV are like sticks of dynamite.
- Another good tip for boys together is to give their need to get physical more of a goal – structured boisterousness rather than random rough and tumble. "Sometimes I feel like one of those American sergeants," says Mark, father of Daniel, 10, Tom, seven, and Rory, five. "If they start to fight or bounce off the walls, I round them up and get them doing star jumps, or doing laps around the garden or up and down the stairs. I give rewards for the fastest ten laps, and make sure they each win something. Or I get them chanting as they jump, or counting, or shouting out things. Anything to distract them and wear them out."

- Encourage boys to be verbal. Talk to him, listen to him – make him feel that expressing feelings is normal and healthy in your home. "We make sure Ben spends time reading with us," says David. "And that leads to conversations. Mandy also makes sure she spends a bit of time talking with him when he gets out of pre-school."

- Realise that boys – from about nine months old – focus more on objects than people. If he's playing with a truck, get a truck of your own and get down on the floor next to him.

- From about 18 months, they get a surge of 'boy energy'. "We put out a lot of soft pillows and tumbling mats on the floor," says Mark. "Then they can wrestle and jump and career about and they don't break our stuff."

- Teach him chores. It's not just about telling him that girls are not just there to clean up after him – it's also about setting him up to be a capable man when he leaves home. Smart men are men who can look after themselves and other people. "My older brother was absolutely hopeless when he went off to college," remembers Amy, mother of Jack, two. "He couldn't even open a tin of beans, or wash his own clothes. He had to learn fast. But I'm determined that Jack will know how to look after himself. Even now, he helps me dust and cook and fold the washed clothes."

- And if he does a household chore well, make sure daddy praises him too. Boys will look to their father to judge what is acceptable. It's vital that dad is seen to cook, shop, wash and so on – as though it's normal for men to do it, rather than saying "We're doing this to help Mummy". Even now, my husband takes pride in ironing his work shirts, because he grew up seeing his own father do that particular chore. Equally, mum should change the odd lightbulb or look under the car bonnet from time to time.

- If your boy is packed with a surge of aggression, try games and role play to help him through it. Read books about boys who are strong and dynamic but also sensitive and kind. Ask him to draw a picture of how he feels inside. Play a game with his favourite action figures having feelings, being afraid, or lonely, and asking their friends to help them. "This actually worked for Joshua when he started school," says Paul. "There was another boy who was making him feel sad. It all came out one evening when he was playing with his Buzz Lightyear, and we ended up making up a game about how Josh could deal with it better. He'd been withdrawn for days, and after that he seemed much happier."

- Also, if he's ripping the heads off his action toys and being aggressive, join in. Rip a head off too. Then say "Oh, no, that was Jack, my best friend. Poor Jack! He must be hurt – let's call the doctors to put his head back on." You've just introduced the ideas of rescue and friendship.

- Give boys short-term goals rather than vague directions. Saying "Let's see if you can pass your maths test next week" will work better than "I really want you to do better at school".

- Hug him. Lots. And kiss him. Let him talk about his fears if he wants to. Tell him that feelings are for humans, not just for girls. Strong boys aren't afraid to tell you what's inside.

Girls with gusto

Best girly tips are:

- Give girls choices. And respect them when they make them – don't force them to be compliant to you. Most women remember being coerced into going round a room full of guests in the evening, offering goodnight kisses to all and sundry. And most women hated it. If your child would prefer to blow a kiss from the door, let her.
- Equally, give her a little privacy as she gets older. Evie, now four, has recently decided that poos will be done in private. I am allowed in at the end to check the wiping. And to be honest, I think that's fair enough – I prefer to poo in private too.
- Don't be afraid to say "No" – firmly, if necessary. Some parents skirt round this with their daughters, indulging them in a way they wouldn't dream of with their sons. But girls need boundaries too, and they need to know you mean it.
- Girls tend to have better language skills earlier than boys, which helps with their verbal self-expression. But encourage her to *do* stuff too – let her get messy, climb trees, jump in puddles. Brains learn by *doing* – it's only by doing

these things that the nervous system can build the necessary pathways in the brain for her to learn. Got a prim princess? Make the fairy castle be *up* the tree, or *across* the muddy puddle, or *through* the plastic tunnel.

- Daddies should beware of their daughters' attempts to wrap them round their little fingers. Small indulgences are the most wonderful part of the daddy–daughter relationship, but teaching her that batting her eyelashes will win her the world won't do her any favours when she grows up.
- Instead, dads can help stretch their daughters' abilities. Don't be too over-protective. If she can't do a puzzle, don't take over – help her to keep trying and find a solution. You want her to be capable, not helpless and dependent.
- Allow girls to show strong feelings, even if those feelings are not pretty. If she's jealous, or furious, or frustrated, let her get those feelings out. Take her to the park and let her yell as loud as she can, or give her a pillow to punch. "We tried this with Olivia," says Piers. "As a child, Victoria remembers always being encouraged to be quiet and keep feelings in check, but we've both made a big effort to let Olivia express whatever she's feeling. Our favourite way is going out with the dog, throwing sticks around and yelling a lot."
- Get tomboys doing at least a little bit of homely stuff so they learn how to look after themselves. Sneaky ways to do this include messy cooking – lots of goo and beating with

a spoon – or washing the car/floor/windows in overalls and waterproofs.

- If you've got a little fairy, let her dress up and paint her nails. But buy the doctor's bag rather than the nurse's one, and ask her if she'd rather create the fashion than just model it. "When Esme said she wanted to be a model, we rolled our eyes," says Peter, whose daughter is nearly four. "But my mother said she'd help her sew a dress to wear. Jackie says she can't even sew on a button, but my mother's great at all that stuff. In the end, they spent hours making things together and now Esme says she's going to be a fashion designer."

In short, you need lots of variety and not too much judgement. Have fun. There's room in the world for all sorts, so try to remember that when your son is shooting the cat, or trying on your lipstick, or your daughter is stealing your best high heels, or knocking ten bells out of the next door neighbour's little girl. When it comes to it, little girls and little boys aren't 'made out of' anything we can control – so stop trying.

CHAPTER 10

Friends

Playmates, play dates and popularity

Last year, my daughter had a 'best friend'. Both Evie and the friend were three years old. At pre-school, their teachers told me, they regularly had quarrels during which they would proclaim dramatically that "You are not my best friend any more!"– only to make up equally dramatically minutes later with emotional hugs and displays of affection.

Naively, I thought this kind of thing only started at 'proper' school. Best friends? Falling out? Wasn't that for when you're about 13?

Apparently not. Girls tend to start all this much earlier than boys, say the teachers. Boys of pre-school age tend to run in packs, all friends together, content to bond over cars and bricks and boy stuff, their only proviso being that Girls Are Not Allowed. Well, not in school, anyway.

Girls, even when they are two or three, can be cliquey. In my daughter's class, there was a very definite division of girls into pairs of friends – at least in my daughter's mind. "Oh yes, Poppy is nice," she would assure me. "But she's best friends with Carrie. They play with us sometimes, but they're mostly just together."

Thankfully, a year on, Evie and her 'best friend' seem to have widened their circle and both they, and the other paired-off girls, although still close, are more willing to be friends with other girls too. But for a while, many of us mums found it disconcerting, if sometimes rather sweet, that even very young toddlers could become so attached to a particular friend.

The up side is that these friendships do teach them skills they can't get from you. Despite their willingness to make friends, at this age they are not mature enough to do all the things that make a complex relationship run smoothly – listen, take turns, see another person's point of view. But through their close friendship, they will learn these things.

Which is all very well, but when your child and their 'best friend' are busy bashing the living daylights out of each other during a row, or ripping apart a coveted toy, you may need a few sneaky shortcuts in hand to help you calm the waters.

Making friends

Firstly, what if yours is the child languishing all on their own in the corner, with not a friend in sight? If that doesn't twist the gut of a parent and take them straight back to playground banishment scenarios themselves, what does?

"When we moved house, Heather started in a nursery where everybody knew everyone else already," says Caroline, whose daughter is now four. "I helped her make friends by saying things like 'Look, that girl has the same shoes/bag/hairband as you,' and that normally initiated conversation. For girls especially, I think that works well. If I know the family has a dog, or rabbit, I might say 'Look, there's Anna, do you know she has a rabbit?' Heather normally then gets excited and talks to Anna about the rabbit."

At this early age, parents can mediate without causing too much embarrassment to a mortified chid. Evie's grandmother Christine, who often looks after Evie's cousin Freddy, three, says: "Freddy is a real loner. At mother and toddler group, he didn't want other children to play with him. If he'd got a truck and another child put their hand on it, he'd move the hand away. So what I did was get the other child involved myself – if there was a jigsaw puzzle, I'd get them playing with it as well as Freddy. Before they knew it, they were doing it together. If I'd just left it to Freddy, it would never have happened."

To achieve the same effect with an older child requires a little more devious thinking. Richard, who has a boy and two girls, often finds that on holiday his daughters club together and his son Oliver, eight, is left out, which means Richard has to stand in as 'mate'. "We often go camping," he says. "I'll target another boy of about the same age and suggest to my son that we have a game of cricket, which just happens to be right outside the other boy's caravan. The boy watches us, and I'll ask if he wants to have a go. So they start playing, and eventually I wander off and leave them to it. The last time I did this, the two boys were friends for the rest of the week."

If you have a child who is very shy, rather than just antisocial in a normal toddler fashion, life can seem very hard work. But forcing a shy child to be social can damage an already fragile self-esteem. "It's so hard when yours is the only child clinging to your leg at a party," says Rob, father of Chloe, four. "We try very hard not to let Chloe hear us describe her as 'shy'. We don't want to give her a label. We just try and boost her confidence, and let her be herself.

"We also found a playgroup where the numbers were small, so it wasn't too intimidating for her, and we invite other children round to play with her on her own turf so she feels confident. Often, if the other children are slightly younger than her, she feels she can take the lead, and is noticeably more outgoing."

Shy children need a little bit more of a guiding hand. But beware being too much of a friendship Machiavelli. Maxine, mother of Evie's cousins Marnie and Freddy, says: "I have definitely noticed that the children of mums who 'get involved' too much – I mean trying to sort out disputes the second they happen, and trying to push their children to play with people that the children don't naturally go to – are less capable of making friends by themselves."

Play dates

The most obvious kind of friendship 'engineering' is the now ubiquitous 'play date'. This concept, which seems to have migrated from America, is in my experience now the standard tool for encouraging social niceties in younger children.

It's scary. Dates are arranged with the smiling ferocity of a society party circuit hostess. Mothers who would not normally have two words to say to each other find themselves putting aside their differences for the sake of developing a socially adept child.

And if you're not careful, even the most meticulously planned play date can end up resembling the War of the Worlds with your children lying wounded in a field of bright plastic shrapnel and toy debris.

"Someone should write a book about play date etiquette," says Mandy, mother of Ben, four. "It's a minefield. I nearly lost a good friend of mine because a play date between my son and her son went horribly wrong. It took us six months to get back to normal."

The play date, above all things, needs a good back-up of sneaky shortcuts:

- To begin with, offer to host the play date at your house. Your child will be on home ground, and you will be there to play United Nations.

- Set out the rules at the start. They might include sharing toys, taking turns, using polite words, no throwing, no hitting or punching, no calling names – decide what's important to you.

- Don't step in like an army major at the first sign of trouble. Let them have a go at sorting out their own disputes. But keep your ears open for any flashpoints where things might get out of hand.

- Set a time limit – two hours is plenty for young children or children who don't know each other very well. "It's good to have a pre-prepared excuse to call an end to it," says Mandy. "When Ben was a bit younger, I always used to say he needed to have his nap. Now, I'll often invent an appointment, or say we need to go and pick Daddy up from the station."
- Choose a time when the children are not tired or hungry. Having a play date straight after a morning pre-school session, for example, is a bad idea.
- Be clever with toys. "Ben puts away any of his very special toys that he doesn't want to share," says Mandy. "Anything that's out has to be shared – that's the deal. And I make sure I get out toys that have more than one component – boxes of cars and trains, or animals. If there's just one big dinosaur, he gets put away."
- Consider going to places where there are no toys to play tug of war with. Playgrounds are great in summer, or beaches. "When the weather's not been good, I've sometimes just put on some music for them in the living room and let them dance around," says Mandy.
- Be creative. Make a den for them on your double bed with a blanket, or go on a nature walk to collect things in a paper bag – experiences are easier to share than objects at this age. "Once, on one rather grim November afternoon, I just plonked Olivia and her friend in the bath," says Victoria, mother of Olivia, three. "The friend's mother was with us and said it was fine. We got out the bath toys

and the bath crayons and they stayed in there quite happily until they were wrinkled."

- Use food as a tool. Once you've asked your child's friend's parent if it's fine to feed them – and checked for allergies – snacks and meals can be a godsend. "A meal helps break up the play time," says Victoria. "It's a fantastic diversion if they're starting to get irritable with each other. Saying 'Who wants a snack?' always works. And if the food is served out on a blanket on the lawn, or even on the carpet, so much the better."

Invisible friends

All this is fine if your child's friend is flesh and bone. But if your child happens to have a friend of the imaginary kind, a few extra sneaky tips might be needed.

Imaginary friends are common at the pre-school age, when children are developing rich and imaginative inner worlds. More common with only or first-born children, they are seen as a normal part of development by child psychologists, and as long as your child is also sociable and outgoing when real children are around, the feeling is that you have nothing to worry about. In fact, children with imaginary friends might be a lot better off than children who have so many toys and such a busy schedule thrust upon them that they have no opportunity to let their imaginations flourish.

Current advice is to let your child have their inner world – don't question them too doggedly about it, or make fun of it.

Play along to an extent – remember the friend's name, apologise when you sit on them – you're showing respect for your child's creation.

Remember, it's a great way for them to practise the social skills they need in real life. And occasionally, that imaginary friend can come in very handy. "We used to tell Esme that her friend, who she called Binks, loved carrots," says Peter. "Binks was responsible for getting our daughter to eat vegetables."

Whatever the nature of your child's friends, be they imaginary or otherwise, you are bound to worry about your child's popularity and ability to mix with their peer group. A lot of your feelings and attitudes may stem from your own memories, good or bad, of friendships you had as a child.

But try not to load your baggage onto your child. The one tip that most mums have to offer is to practise the art of gritting your teeth and saying nothing while pasting on a bright friendly smile – and letting your child learn how to be a good friend the hard way.

CHAPTER 11

Siblings

From new baby envy to rampant sibling rivalry: how to maintain the peace

If you think trying to get your child to play peacefully with their friends is a task and a half, wait until they have a sibling. Rare is the parent who has told me that their children exist in a harmonious bubble of sibling friendship, with only the most minor of squabbles to sort out.

For the majority of parents with more than one child, it seems, sibling rivalry requires graduation to the very highest level of family diplomacy – and sneakiness.

I write as a parent who is only just stepping up onto this challenging rung of the parenting ladder. Evie's baby brother Charlie has just arrived, and we have only had a few weeks of coping with a sibling who is all too loud and apparent in our home, as opposed to one safely inside me, where only the strongest of pokes from an interested sisterly finger could disturb his peace.

So forgive me if I rely heavily on other parents and sibling warfare experts to guide me through this chapter – although I can talk with some authority on how to tell a three year old that they are soon to be a big sister.

In fact, that's where we'll start – how to prepare a child for the arrival of a new sibling. My feeling is that this will be greatly influenced by whether or not you decide to find out the baby's gender before the birth.

If you prefer to wait for a surprise, then the concept of 'the new baby' will be somewhat vague to your child, which some parents might think is an advantage. The blunt reality of a rival for your time and affection will come soon enough.

We found out at 20 weeks that we were expecting a boy. This came in handy in two respects – firstly, I had time to console a disappointed Evie who was desperate for a baby sister called Daisy but who, in time, came round to the fact that she would have a baby brother (although she'd still have preferred him to be called Daisy); secondly, that she was able to 'bond' with her future brother, and even when he was still in the womb, she readily referred to 'him' and what he would be like, where he would sleep, how she would help bathe him and play with him and so on.

Finding out in advance definitely gives you time for a PR assault on your existing child; we were able to barrage Evie with a list of good things about baby brothers – Peppa Pig has one; so does her idolised big cousin Marnie; a baby brother might not be quite so keen to play with all her pink fairy toys (this was the clincher). Within two weeks she was as excited about his arrival as we were.

The arrival

Whatever you choose, and whatever the variety of sibling to

come, there are a few shortcuts to making their arrival go smoothly:

- Prepare your child by letting them touch the bump, kiss it, talk to the baby and so on, and get involved in baby preparations. "To prepare Heather (four) for Murray, we told her early on and made a joke of my tummy as it got bigger," says Caroline. "I let her talk to the bump and we made a silly voice to reply to her which we carried on when he was born. She helped decorate his room, and put the toys out. We let her help choose new baby outfits. And we let her play with all the old and new baby stuff – her old pram, baby slings, rattles, Moses basket – before he came on the scene. I often found her pretending with her dolls that it was her baby, and it helped that the novelty factor wore off before we actually needed all the equipment."
- Also prepare them for the reality. Tell them that mummy will need to hold and carry the baby a lot, and will have to cuddle it when it cries. "We explained that the baby would cry a lot, and boy did he cry!" says Caroline. "Also, we would talk to her as an equal once Murray was here. 'Wasn't Murray noisy last night! Did he keep you awake?' or 'Isn't Murray's crying really piercing? It must be difficult for you to hear the TV,' which I think she really appreciated."
- Talk about 'us' and 'the baby', so you align your child with yourself as 'one of us', advises Roni, mother of Jack, now 10, Ned, eight, and Hal, five. "Say 'We're going to have to

teach the baby to smile,' or 'The baby will love getting cuddles from us,'" says Roni. "This helps your child feel closer to you, and part of the team."

- Let your child know you remember when they were a baby, and how special it was too. Look through their baby photo album with them. We even got out Evie's very first ultrasound scan photos and compared them to the ones of the new baby. And by seeing pictures of themselves at an early stage, they will be more prepared for what will happen with their brother or sister.
- Have a present ready for your older child 'from' the baby when they first come to visit at the hospital. Nic, mother of Liam, four, and baby Kieran, remembers: "The first time Liam visited us in hospital there was a present waiting for him. Also, on the way in, Hugh and Liam stopped at the shop and Liam was allowed to choose a present for Kieran. He bought a balloon which we tied to the cot. We also made sure that, apart from the day I had my Caesarean, Liam wasn't left at home while Hugh visited the hospital. We didn't want him to feel left out at all. Liam loved it – he would do little jobs for me such as filling my water bottle and collecting my lunch. His favourite part was watching the TV at the side of my bed – he still talks about it now."
- Older children can obviously get even more involved. Marnie, Evie's cousin, was six when her little brother Freddy came along. "She watched the video we had done at the 12-week scan, and came with me to midwife

appointments, where she listened to the heartbeat," says Maxine. "She was one of the few 'only child' families in her school class, so she was quite ready to extend our family. And the school helped too – she used to tell the teacher about waiting for the baby, and they made a fuss about it which made Marnie feel special."

- And even older children aren't too big for presents. "We gave Marnie a card from her new brother with a big rosette on the front saying 'I'm a big sister', and gave her a present from Freddy which didn't fool her for a minute, but she was still pleased." says Maxine. "The thing she was most desperate for was to take the baby to her school to show him off, so we did that as soon as possible."
- "We made Josh and Arthur their own 'big brother' baskets which they got at the hospital on the day Mabel was born," says Paul. "They had crayons and a colouring book for Arthur, a robot thing for Josh, snacks, drinks and that sort of thing in them – and a card saying 'From your new little sister'. It kept them amused, and made them feel special."
- When you bring the baby home, have daddy carry it into the house for a first time, so mummy's hands are free for a cuddle.
- If you are comfortable with the idea of a home birth – statistically at least as safe as a hospital birth – this can be the best option for your older child or children, as you don't go away and leave them at all. They are part of the whole birth process.

- Expect lots of visitors bearing gifts. Sensitive ones, and clued up parents, will bring a small one for your older child too – but perhaps have a stash of cheap toys somewhere so your child isn't left out when you're opening a baby gift.
- Make the birth a celebration. "Melanie bought a frozen cake in advance, and when she and Mabel got home, I just defrosted it and we had a simple 'birthday party' with ice cream and hats for the boys," says Paul. "It actually kept them happy while Mel got settled in with the baby."

Settling in

Once the baby is home, it is natural to have a bit of a panic over how one parent with one pair of hands can divide themselves between two or more children. "I used to get stressed about how I would cope with two demanding my attention at the same time, but it never really came to be a problem," says Caroline. "If Heather needed something, I would just stop what I was doing and sort her out with a toilet trip, drink, toy or whatever because Murray was too young to realise what was happening."

Sneaky attention-dividing shortcuts include:

- Getting the older child involved. Some really respond to being Mother's Helper. "We allowed Heather to hold Murray, wash him, and change his nappy (with supervision)," says Caroline. "We also made her run errands for which she got lots of praise – fetching nappies, a towel, helping me bathe him. She was actually really helpful."

- Finding creative ways to reassure yourself. "A funny thing that sticks in my mind from the first few days of being alone with Liam and Kieran is that each morning I'd find I needed to go to the toilet, but I was nervous of leaving them on their own and it seemed a lot of hassle to take Kieran with me," says Nic. "As it was usually around breakfast time, I'd fill Liam's bowl with his favourite cereal – and as long as I could hear his spoon hitting the bowl, I knew that Kieran was safe."

- Spending as much time as you can sitting on the floor with your baby in your arms. It makes you more accessible to your other child. Slings are also good for freeing up parental arms. As the baby gets older, use an infant seat or put them on a blanket to watch you play with their older brother and sister.

- Averting over-zealous "attention". "We put Daisy in her Moses basket or her recliner inside a playpen if we had to leave the room for a few seconds," says Jess, also mother of Molly, three. "It meant a very inquisitive Molly couldn't accidentally hurt Daisy because she could see her, but not reach her."

- Using daddy, a partner or a grandparent to shower the older sibling with extra attention, trips and adventures. Make up for your distraction with extra 'special' time with other family members.

- Being tactful. If an admirer gushes about your baby within earshot of your other child, say something like "Yes, now we have two gorgeous children!"

- Being prepared for regression, even in an apparently happy older sibling. When they realise the baby's here for ever – or when the baby starts crawling and can get into their things – many children regress to wanting dummies and nappies, wetting themselves, wanting to be fed or sleep in a cot, or speaking in a baby voice. One friend remembers an acquaintance telling her of a particularly bad day at a Tumble Tots session when her elder boy, in an attempt to distract her from breastfeeding her new baby, began weeing and pooing on the floor in front of everybody. The mother confessed to leaving both children in the class, running out of the front door wailing "Take them! Take them both!" She hasn't, I am told, been back since.

- "We tried to ignore it," says Paul of the regression issue. "When Mabel came along, Arthur was two and just out of nappies, but that all went wrong again. He used to say he wanted to be a baby, but when he realised that meant he couldn't play on his trike or eat his favourite banana sandwiches, he quickly changed his mind."

- Trying not to blame everything on *the baby*. Rather than saying "Be quiet, the baby's sleeping," or "You've made the baby cry," say "See how quietly you can whisper for a while," or "What can we think of to do that will make the baby happy again?"

- Starting the day, whenever you can, with just a few minutes of 'special time' with your older child. A few minutes of cuddles and listening can ward off angry feelings towards a new arrival, and set them up positively for the rest of the day.

Sibling soothers

Once you've got through the initial new baby stage, things can actually seem harder – the novelty has worn off, and now you have a lifetime of peace negotiations to contemplate. Apparently children spend about a third of their free time with their siblings, so it's no wonder that all that proximity can create problems. Soothing sibling squabbles requires a sneaky – but subtle – approach. The aim: to have your children think any goodwill or affection they show to each other is *their* idea, or *their* initiative, and that you hadn't even noticed the slightest tension in the house.

top tips

A few more tips for happy sibling relationships:

- Don't stress about the small things. "We let the children sort out little squabbles over toys by themselves," says Paul, who is a veteran peacemaker with eight year old son Joshua as well as Arthur, five, and Mabel, three. "We just say something like 'If you haven't worked it out in five minutes, the toy goes in the shed'. We only step in when there is hitting, or name calling, or one of them is feeling bullied by the others."
- Don't take sides, or encourage them to tell tales. If there's an argument, send both to their rooms, whoever started it. Even if it's obvious who's at fault, be sneakily dim – pretend you didn't see.
- Create a 'time out' space for toys. "We have a toy 'jail' on top

of a cupboard in our kitchen," says Paul. "If they fight over something small, it goes to jail. If it's something big, it goes in the shed."

- Encourage siblings to be compassionate towards each other. Ask one to help tend to another's injury, such as a grazed knee. "We will sometimes ask Arthur to hold Mabel's leg while we put cream on a graze," says Dave. "It helps him feel tender towards her, and she's less likely to taunt him if he's been kind."
- Let older children share their skills. "We got Josh, who loves football, to teach Arthur how to kick a ball," says Paul. "In fact, he ended up teaching Mabel as well."

Don't worry too much about that old aim of treating children 'equally'. Yes, they will keep score and test you about who you love more. Paul and Melanie's younger two even kept count of pieces of roast potato on the plate one Sunday lunchtime to make sure they got an equal number. But reassure them that you love them all in special ways. "We tell ours that it's like flowers in the sun – having more flowers doesn't mean each one gets less sun," says Melanie. What they want is to be treated as individuals, not equals.

Depending on their age gaps, personalities and background, your children could carry on competing right through early childhood toys, school day exam grades and teenage friends. They might even still be doing it as adults. So it's important to stay calm and save your energy for the long haul.

The best thing you can teach them right from the beginning

is that, one day, they'll realise that their brothers and sisters will become their best friends. Other friends may come and go but, whatever their differences, siblings are forever.

CHAPTER 12

Relative values

The modern grandparent and how to operate one

Families these days are entities which are rather difficult to define. They come in all shapes and sizes. Also, they are undergoing enormous change – not many of us still live in a village with most of our living relatives within a five-mile radius, providing an ever-constant comfort blanket of help, advice and continuity.

Modern-day grandparents range from those who communicate with their grandchildren by webcam across a continent, to those who look after their grandchildren full-time while their children go back to work. And anything in between.

Families are in their most flexible and diverse state ever. They have to be. And yet, it still can seem so hard to get the balance right. How is it that our parents, the people we often love the most and the family with whom our children will usually have the closest contact, can sometimes be so challenging?

It seems to me that, were you to receive an instruction manual with every grandparent, there would be three main models:

- The traditional grandparents – on hand for weekend visits and treats.
- Grandparents who are practically stand-in parents.
- Grandparents who would rather undergo Japanese water torture than go anywhere near a nappy or, for that matter, any child under the age of 15.

Add to this the variation of whether the grandparent in question is on your side of the family or on your partner's side.

If the grandparent is 'yours', there may be long-standing issues, baggage, family rows; if the grandparent is an in-law, there is potential for clashes of personality, competition, perceived criticism. So, a veritable melting pot of inter-generational sensitivities to contend with.

Luckily, most of us will end up with the first model – fun visits and occasional treats. But a few will recognise that they have 'models' at the extreme ends of the scale.

All-singing, all-dancing grandparents

Christine is Evie's grandmother on her daddy's side. She looks after Evie's cousins Marnie, nine, and Freddy, three, while their mother Maxine works full-time. A pretty hands-on grandparent, by any standards. But this kind of arrangement takes a fair bit of sneaky management:

- Keep a sense of humour if your children sometimes seem to think Grandma is more appealing than you. "Where

Maxine is so good is that she trusts me completely – even if I butt in when she's there," says Christine. "One day, Freddy even pushed her out of my front door with a 'No Mummy!' because he knew it was our time to play together after pre-school, but she was laughing, calling through the letterbox. She wasn't hurt – she loves my relationship with her children."

- Let your parent or parent-in-law be the 'fun nanny' or 'fun grandad' sometimes, and not just the carer. "If you're there all the time, sometimes you feel the grandchildren don't have that excitement they feel towards their other grandmother," says Christine. "But I make sure I sometimes do special things, like take Marnie to the pictures or to a show, so we can have a treat together."

Barbara's children, Kate and Victoria, now grown up, always had a very close relationship with Barbara's parents, who were extremely hands-on while Barbara was studying and the children were young. "It meant that they really bonded, which I loved," Barbara recalls. "But it can be hard when your parents have diverse ideas about things like discipline. If one thinks that if you love children enough, they don't need discipline, and the other is much more strict, you can end up confused, veering between the two and giving a mixed message. You have to try to have the courage of your own convictions. But it's hard to say 'Could you please just help with the washing, set the table and fold the nappies and leave the parenting to me' when you so badly need – and appreciate – their help."

If your children's grandparents get too involved in enforcing the rules, you could try the 'Parents are for discipline, grandparents are for spoiling' mantra. But what do you do if spoiling is the problem? Do your children come home from visits to their grandparents tanked up on sugar and bearing the entire contents of the local toy shop? And if so, what do you do?

"My mother-in-law knows that if she doesn't follow the rules, she won't get babysitting privileges," says Mark, father of Daniel, 10, Tom, seven, and Rory, five. "She really wants to be involved in their lives, so she behaves herself. We've also worked out other ways of 'spoiling,' like extra trips out instead of sweets and toys."

If you're struggling to draw lines between what you and your very enthusiastic parents do with your children, one tip is to find a niche for them to fill that doesn't tread on your toes. Do they like gardening, and you hate it? Get the children out there with them creating a vegetable patch, or growing sunflowers. Does your mother-in-law love to bake but your cookbooks went AWOL years ago? Let her do the fairy cakes for your daughter's next school fete. At least you won't have to stay up the night before doctoring shop-bought fairy cakes with home-made icing to make them look authentic. Like I did recently – with the shame only a 'fairy cake fraud' can feel.

The reluctant grandparent

Caroline, mother of Heather, four, and baby Murray, lives in the same village as her mother. She lost her father to cancer.

"I always imagined what a granny should be, and deep down I think that we all want the granny baking in the rose-covered cottage telling stories and making jam, but how often does that happen?" she says.

"My mother openly hates children under the age of six. By the age of one, Murray had met my mum at the most 10 times. She lives half a mile away from us. She will not babysit on her own, or at night, or really at any time if she can possibly help it. When Murray was five months old, Heather pulled an ornament onto her head and I had to take her to hospital. It was 10am and my mother wouldn't come to watch Murray because she was still in bed. No discussion, that's just how she is.

"Even when I was about to have Murray, a week overdue, she wouldn't come to look after Heather while I went to the hospital to be assessed. She said: 'No, could you not have planned this a bit better?' It was 11am, but she said she had to catch up on some TV she'd recorded the night before. Heather had to go to a neighbour, and I went into labour driving myself to the hospital."

Caroline adds: "My mother-in-law is a doddle by comparison. She has some strong views – potty training should be complete by the age of 12 months, babies love a wee drink of tea, spanking should be mandatory – but the difference is the amount of time she and my father-in-law devote to Heather and Murray. Endless games of jigsaws, chase in the garden, baking with grandma. But they are a bit nervous – they see their fellow grandparent friends caring for their grandchildren several days a week, and how this takes over their lives, and are a bit worried I'm going to announce I'm going back to work."

top tips

Caroline's top tips:

- Settle for what you've got and get on with it. Heather thinks the world of my mum, despite the difficulties – so I remind myself that despite what I think, there must be something good happening.
- Don't try to change them. My mother did say she would never change a nappy, and she hasn't – at least she's been consistent. Nothing would have made any difference, and sometimes battles are just not worth getting into. Maybe they can offer something else that your child will love them for.

Other operating instructions

Whether the grandparents in your family are at the extreme ends of the scale or are rather more middle-of-the-road, there are always a few smart shortcuts to harmonious grandparenting. Call them the Grandparent Charter:

- Lay down your ground rules. Let your parents, or parents-in-law, know which are the 'big issues' for you.
- Then pick your battles. Don't expect them to care for your child in a straitjacket made of your own rules. Stick to the big stuff.
- Don't worry too much if some rules are relaxed at nanny's

house. Children realise that the things they do with their grandparents are special, and different, and don't expect things to be the same when they return home.

- Don't argue about child-rearing issues in front of the children. Save it for later.
- Don't fly off the handle if they criticise you. Parenting styles change between generations – focus on the things that remain constant, like love and affection.
- Help your children to see their grandparents as 'whole' people. Ask your grandparents to get out their old photos so your children can see what they were like when they were young. Older children could even put together a simple family tree, with drawings and photos. Do it together – you might find out a bit more too.

And finally, remember that the best thing grandparents can offer is time. It doesn't matter how much money they have, or how fancy their garden is, or how outmoded their ideas may be – the time they can give to your child is the most precious thing. "The best times are when you are doing something simple, like collecting shells on the beach, or finding treasures in the garden, and they start to chat to you," says Annie, Evie's maternal grandmother. "Unconditional love, lots of time, and sometimes being a little bit conspiratorial with them – those are the things that count," she says. "That's where the magic is."

CHAPTER 13

Learning

Throw away those flashcards

Everyone thinks their child will be a genius. You may dream of a Premiership striker, a prima ballerina, a Nobel prize-winning scientist or the next poet laureate – we've all got our secret wishes for our offspring. And an absolute conviction that our child is the smartest one we know. Without dispute.

We place value on different things. Being journalists by trade – and therefore 'wordy' but rather hopeless at all things mathematical – my husband and I place verbal skills near the top of our list, and were delighted when Evie proved to be an early, and sometimes rather disconcertingly articulate, talker with a talent for mimicry. How proud we were when she declared, matter-of-factly, at the age of two: "That window is transparent, Mummy." And how shocked when a little voice uttered a perfectly pitched profanity with resigned disgust from the back seat of the car when I stalled it. Oh, the shame.

Others prize physical skills, or a second language at an early age, or musical ability, or flair for painting. Whatever – we want our children to reflect our own coveted abilities. And it's a hard thing sometimes not to give our babies a hefty push in the 'right' direction.

It starts from day one. No – it starts from about minus seven or eight months. Because the minute parents-to-be get to grips with the good news, the barrage starts: 'How to create a genius in the womb,' 'Communicate with your unborn baby,' 'Mozart for fetuses.' From magazine articles to books, CDs, DVDs and websites, they target you accusingly: if your baby is not the smartest child on the block by the time it is born, it will be *your fault*.

With Evie, I remember spending a small fortune on a device that you strap to your bump which enables you not only to hear the baby's heartbeat, but also to play music that they will then recognise and miraculously 'calm down' to when they are a colicky, sleepless newborn. Not only could I only ever make out white noise from the device – and no heartbeat – but I imagine that my attempts to play a bit of gentle, refined Bach twice a day for six months in the womb had little effect either – judging by the fact that her favourite 'going to sleep' songs as a baby were anything by Billy Bragg, and the more militant the better.

After the birth, the pressure steps up. You've only got to watch Child of Our Time or, worse, one of those American documentaries about toddler hot-housing, to get a serious dose of guilt that you haven't spent the first six months of your child's life whipping flashcards in front of their eyes, teaching them baby sign language or buying exactly the right type of stimulating black-and-white cot mobile.

And by the time you have a toddler or pre-schooler, you have probably already succumbed to some extent to that most smugly competitive of pursuits: the 'Which clubs and classes does your child attend?' knock-out contest. Tiny tots' ballet? I'll trump that with Suzuki violin. Tennis for tots? Not a patch on advanced French for the under-fives. Ha!

Home help

Exactly how useful is all that extra-curricular learning? Does it make your child shine at pre-school, and give them a better start in life? Is it a case of 'the more, the better,' or are children likely to be just as bright and happy if they are left, at least some of their time, to learn and develop at their own pace?

Most parents seem to agree that it's a case of 'everything in moderation'. A few classes here and there probably stimulate your child wonderfully, and help them expand their horizons and make new friends. A fully packed timetable of 'educational' pursuits enforced by a highly competitive and demanding parent will probably just lead to a bad case of burn-out and, possibly, a trip to the therapist.

So how can parents take smart shortcuts to learning at home – without all the pressure?

"Everything you do can be 'learning'," says Evie's grandmother Annie. "At that early age, it's all about imagination. They have such amazing internal, imaginative worlds, and if you can enter that with them, you can make the most of it to help them learn. But you've got to do it with them – see what they are naturally learning at that moment, let them take you there and then help them take it just that little bit further."

Which doesn't mean hiring a maths tutor or spending a fortune on specialist DVDs. It means time, and everyday activities.

top tips

Here are a few more tips:

- Count everything. "Biscuits on a plate, pieces of cereal, tins on a shelf, place mats, lamp posts, steps, doors – everything." says David, father of Ben, four. "It soon sinks in."
- From the age of about two, make comparisons. Talk about whose shoes are larger, which cat is hairier, which saucepan holds more soup, which shopping bag weighs more. "We also arrange cupboard stuff from smallest to largest when we're putting away the shopping," says David.
- Make routine things a fun learning time. "Bath time is physics," says Annie. "How much water will fit in this pot? How does it come out through the holes? Does water go uphill? What toys float? A complete lesson in one bath tub."
- Equally, the kitchen is the perfect place for fun lessons. Let your child help you cook. "I have a lovely old-fashioned set of scales with weights, which are great for learning about weighing things," says Annie. "Even making sandwiches for tea can involve different shapes – triangles, squares, circles – and different colours."
- Let them really get stuck in in the kitchen. Evie's daddy regularly has a 'little helper' beside him when he cooks. As a result, Evie knows all about different vegetables, how to pick the freshest ones in the shop, what they smell like, how they

grow, and how they change through cooking. She loves being daddy's commis chef.

- Even the washing up can be a learning experience. Most toddlers love rolling up their sleeves and helping wash up the less breakable objects in your kitchen. At toddler group, I used to help wash up the coffee mugs because Evie often preferred being out in the kitchen with a dishcloth in her hand to playing with toys in the main room.

Making it real

Remember, you as a parent have to be canny. The people who sell flashy educational products, programmes and techniques are doing just that – selling. There is not a great deal of evidence that any particular programmes make a real difference to brain development – and in fact, a recent study even found that children with too many expensive toys were less able to use their imaginations, because they hadn't learned how.

So, if you love Mozart and want to share it with your child, fine. But you could just as well play Westlife or Robbie Williams. Music stimulates, but there is no evidence that certain types of music increase intelligence or will turn your child into a budding physicist.

As for flashcards, this kind of learning is memorising. It's an impressive trick to show off to your friends, but it's not real learning. Children need to learn in context – which means in a 'real' environment.

So, if you're determined that your child will learn to read before they start school, don't force it – have fun with it. Have them read letters and signs in the street, on food tins, on cereal packets, and around the house.

Above all, get out there with them into the 'real world':

- Your own garden, however small, is as educational as any exotic location. "Go on a field trip to your garden and collect things," says Annie. "Watch things grow, listen to the insects." And make them think. Ask them how they think it would feel to be the size of an ant – what would look different, what could you hear and see, what would you be afraid of? What if you were a wasp, and could fly up high and look down on your house?

- Let them make things with their hands. Can they make instruments from sticks, stones, leaves, the watering can? Can they make garden music?

- Engage their senses. Lie on a blanket outside, close your eyes, and ask them what they can hear. Or cut a hole in an old cardboard box, let them put their hand in the hole to feel a household object, and get them to guess what it is by touch alone.

- "I definitely feel that it's better to 'do' the real thing rather than see it on TV or on a DVD," says Caroline, mother of Heather, four, and Murray, one. "Our favourite thing is to talk about the weather, and when it's really windy or wet, to go and stand in it and get absolutely blown about or soaked to the skin. We also love to play with smells – flowers in the garden, smelly cows in the field, spices in the kitchen. What's nice, what's not?"

- Many children, and adults, learn better if they write things down. Young children can do this by drawing – learn the months of the year, for example, by creating a calendar with a drawing for each month: Easter eggs for April, or a bucket and spade for August.

- If something interests you, share it with them. They will learn through your enthusiasm. "David loves old steam trains," says Mandy. "He took Ben to one of those train museums where they dress the trains up as the characters from Thomas the Tank Engine. It sparked a real interest, and now he knows all about how steam engines work."

- Keep their books where they can reach them – on a low book case, or low shelves. Let them choose their own bedtime stories. Sometimes, ask them to 'read' to you – I was amazed the first time I did this that Evie could practically recite the whole story, just using the pictures as reminders. "And don't be afraid to digress from the actual story," says Mandy. "Say things like 'What do you think would have happened if Teddy hadn't been at home? What would his friends have done?'"

Smart shortcuts, when it comes to learning, are not the obvious kind. Fancy things that you just plonk your child in front of may seem like impressive ways to aid intelligence, but all they really are are shortcuts to circus tricks.

The really smart stuff that helps children learn – whether

they be babies, toddlers, pre-schoolers or older – is your time and involvement. The sneaky thing is not to let them catch you 'teaching' them. Watch them, listen to their chatting, get down on their level, and join in. To quote Annie again: "You can't push learning in, with young children. You have to draw it out."

CHAPTER 14

Arty stuff

Play-Doh skills for the manually impaired – or how to create DIY diversions from nothing

Are you someone who saves egg boxes and yoghurt pots for rainy days, knows the perfect recipe for home-made play dough off by heart, and remembers with a warm glowing feeling those Blue Peter 'Here's one I made earlier' creations of your childhood?

Or do you just pop to the nearest toy shop for bulk buys of ready-made craft supplies and ensure that the only time your child comes anywhere near a glue pot or an easel is when they are safely wrapped from head to toe in industrial strength aprons – and preferably on somebody else's premises?

I really wish I were the former. There were people like that at Evie's mother and toddler group, and I have been known to gape in awe as they mentioned in passing their latest craft triumph, and nurture a sizeable inferiority complex as I imagined how much more stimulated, creative and, well, somehow *wholesome* their children must be.

Sadly, I probably veer towards the latter. With occasional, hearty stabs at turning myself, and my daughter, into craft enthusiasts. Evie always loves it when I do, finally, let her get stuck into something good and messy. She's usually slightly bemused, but she loves it.

So if you're already an arty stuff expert, you probably don't need to read this chapter. But if you're of anything less than Blue Peter standard, you might find the following sneaky shortcuts, garnered from various smart if artily challenged parents including two grandmothers and one very imaginative childminder (Nikki), helpful. Or just plain aggravating, depending on your state of mind.

The criteria are that the activities have to be simple, cannot require too many 'ingredients' that have to be bought specially, and are quick to set up. If you want fancy art projects, there are lots of great books available which take you step-by-step through various ideas. But these are sneaky shortcuts for people with time to fill and limited patience.

Fresh air fun

First of all, activities for the garden or, at least, not too far from home. These are perfect for long summer days when it's just too hot to venture out onto the motorways in search of complicated days out:

- Water painting. This one came up over and over again. Use a squeezy bottle such as an empty washing-up liquid bottle, or just a bucket and some paint brushes. Fill with water, and let them 'paint' the outside wall of your house, or the driveway, or the patio. Has to be done on a dry day, obviously. Keeps them amused for hours, and absolutely no mess because it evaporates.

- A variation is to use chalks. Washes off in the rain, or with a squirt from a hosepipe.
- 'Collect and stick': give your child a bag or small bucket to go out into the garden – or further afield if you can go too – and collect 'interesting stuff'. Make a rule: no rubbish, nothing still alive. Then come home and stick it onto card or paper for a collage. This is Evie's favourite garden activity.
- Vary this by sending older children out with a 'to find' list.
- Born-again hippies can use old T-shirts or pillowcases to create tie-dye masterpieces with a bucket of water, some cold water dye and fixative.
- Keep old cardboard boxes to turn into houses, dens, cars and boats with the help of some felt-tip pens or paints out on the lawn.
- If you have a large window or sliding door, providing it's got safety glass, cover it with soap/suds and let your child rub patterns into it with their hands. Can easily be wiped down when they're finished, and leaves you with a nice clean window.

"My sneaky tip is to get the children outside if at all possible," says Melanie, mother of Joshua, eight, Arthur, five, and Mabel, three. "Because I don't think I've ever heard any of our three say the words 'Mum, I'm bored!' when they're outside. Even if it's raining, ours love going out for a charge around in the puddles with wellies and raincoats on. Remember – children actually like getting wet and dirty."

Indoor ideas

If the weather's really too cold or nasty for outside activities, there is plenty you can do inside. Firstly, here are some old favourites and some new ideas using kitchen cupboard staples:

- Cut up old egg boxes and tape the 'humps' together to make animals such as a caterpillar. Cut boxes in half and stick together again lengthways, paint and stick on a paper 'tongue' for a Chinese dragon.
- Use round paper coffee filters to make flowers. Fold filter in half three times. Put some food colouring into a bowl of water, and dip the tip of the filter in. Repeat with a different colour for each 'corner'. Then unfold and lie flat to dry. When dry, twist at the centre and pull into a flower shape. Use pipe cleaners for a stem, and maybe even spritz with your perfume to make a flower smell.
- An old kitchen cupboard favourite: pasta pictures. Use a variety of dried pasta shapes, add glue, and let the fun begin.
- Icing pens (from the supermarket) are great for decorating plain digestive biscuits.
- Pour some paint into an old baking tray and show your

child how to drag string through it and then onto paper to make patterns. Attach a clothes peg to the end of the string to avoid gunky fingers.

- Save the top half of egg boxes, paint, and fill with tissue paper to create Easter nests. Add yellow chicks and chocolate eggs.
- Make paper plate 'masks' – cut into the shape of an animal's head such as a cat, or a chick, or a lion, then paint and tie on elastic.
- Stick a paper doily onto a piece of paper, let your child paint over it, then remove to reveal the pattern underneath.
- Stick halved cocktail sticks (cut off the sharp points) into a lump of modelling clay. Add eyes to make a hedgehog. Then let your child gather leaves to put into an empty ice cream carton for a hedgehog nest.
- An old favourite: cut vegetables such as potatoes in half and make a simple shape into the cut surface. Dip into paint and push down on paper to make a pattern.
- Use pots, pans and wooden spoons for an impromptu 'concert'. Ear plugs optional.
- A sink full of water, some washing-up liquid and a whisk can entertain for hours. "Don't underrate the ordinary," says Evie's Nannie Annie. "Even better, try hand-washing dollies' clothes, then hanging them up to dry with pegs. And then pretend ironing – it can last all afternoon."

- Take any jars and containers of food you have in the fridge, or the herbs and spices in your spice rack. Open them one at a time and let your child smell them with their eyes shut – let them guess the ingredient. Also talk about colours, smells, tastes. Some ingredients can then be used to create a 'taste painting'.

- Home-made play dough. As mentioned, this isn't the place for detailed recipes and projects, but I have to make an exception for this craft staple. This recipe comes from Evie's Nanny Chris. By the way, garlic presses and cookie cutters make great modelling implements.

Play dough

Ingredients

2 tablespoons cooking oil

2 cups plain flour

1 cup salt

1 cup water

2 teaspoons cream of tartar

Few drops of food colouring

Method

Add the food colouring to the water, then mix all the ingredients together in a large saucepan. Cook on a medium heat, stirring all the time, until the mixture leaves the sides. Cover with a damp towel to cool a little, then knead well – don't burn your hands by doing it too soon. Leave to cool, and store in an airtight container.

"They love actually making the clay, with some careful

> supervision, before they've even started playing with it," says Christine. "So you get double value. This recipe really makes the most pliable stuff to roll out – it's much better than the stuff you buy."

"We used to spend an absolute fortune on craft stuff for Chloe," says Rob, whose daughter is four. "And usually the kits ended up being too fiddly for her even to concentrate on, so we often didn't finish them. I think we just didn't have the confidence to do it ourselves. Now, we use more ordinary household stuff. It keeps her interested for longer, and is much cheaper. It doesn't have to be a perfect creation – just cover everything with a plastic cover and let them at it."

Get creative

Sneaky parents can make everyday or discarded objects and familiar situations turn magically into something fun.

top tips

Here are soome tips for using everyday objects:

- Use old photos that weren't good enough for your albums, and old birthday cards, to cut up and make collages, or give them an old empty album so they can design their own album.
- Use old/spare ceramic wall tiles to make hand or foot prints of your child on with paint. Write their name at the bottom, and seal with varnish after 24 hours.

- Keep a 'boredom box' with leftover ribbons, tags from gifts, paste jewellery, buttons, pebbles, feathers, glitter, magazines and catalogues for cutting out. "Olivia thinks this is her 'treasure' and it will keep her amused for hours," says Victoria.
- Use a digital camera to zoom in close on familiar objects around the house. Print out, and use for an inside treasure hunt.
- If you have an office at home, try letting your child 'Go to work'. Use safe office supplies such as pens, paper and supervised hole punches, and let them put things into a ring binder.
- Create a home cinema – get your child to choose a DVD and then make posters, tickets and popcorn. "Great for family gatherings or when friends come round too," says Anji, mother of Callum, three.
- Create a Family History Box. "Evie and I are going to collect old photos, scraps and stories about our family and collect them to put into a scrapbook," says Annie. "Children love to hear family tales."
- Grow an 'indoor garden' with cress – add pine cones, clay creatures, toy figures etc to make little worlds to fire their imaginations.

"This kind of thing is the sort of activity which makes you feel really pleased with yourself: 'I am a great mum after all!'" says Anji, mother of Callum, three, and provider of the home cinema idea. "Usually I am just too tired or unimaginative to do things which need preparation. But when I do, they really work. And they're also great for only children and getting them to interact when they have a friend round – they really get them playing well together."

After all those ideas, you may find you have an over-abundance of creative masterpieces to find room for in your house. Space-saving ideas include letting your child help select their favourite pieces, and stick them in a scrap book or a large artwork display folder, available from discount stationery stores. Or simply take a photo of the creations and stick the photos in an album or save on your computer in a file marked 'Work of a Mini Genius'.

And if all of this has left you feeling slightly dizzy with creative block, don't worry. Most of us only get around to one or two of these activities per year. Be selective – or use as an ideas list to send with them when they go to stay with grandma.

CHAPTER 15

Equipment

Toddler kit and what you don't need

As first-time parents, it's understandable that you get sucked in by the excitement of it all: you leaf through nursery catalogues, wide-eyed at all the amazing gadgets and cute accessories you never realised you just had to have. After all, if they say you need it, it's a must, right?

And so you buy. And buy some more. And at least a third of the things you buy are still languishing, practically unused and sometimes even unwrapped, at the back of the cupboard, or under the bed, or in the boot of the car, three years later.

Of course, parents doing the whole new baby and toddler thing for the second – or more – time around are completely savvy, know exactly what they will need and what not, and don't spend a penny more on purchases than is strictly necessary. Or … not.

Very much not, if I am anything to go by. Recently pregnant with my second child, I had an extremely hard time controlling my nest-feathering instincts. Yes, I probably did have a much better idea of what equipment is actually helpful and what is merely a ploy to empty the pockets of enthusiastic parents. But despite this, was I actually any better at not buying all the gorgeous goodies on offer? No. And to make matters worse, this time it was a boy, so I was using the excuse that half of Evie's pink and frilly kit just *would not do*, and that new blue boyish gear was the only way to go.

However, I did try hard to listen to the advice of my more experienced parent friends, and filter out the more outstandingly money-wasting, or inconvenient, or just plain inefficient items. It's a rather subjective topic, as some people will swear by a product that others have absolutely no time for. But, before you buy up the entire contents of your nearest nursery stockist in one fell swoop, it might be worth casting your eye over some top tips from people who have been there and lived to recycle their baby baths.

Money savers

Before we get down to details, a few general shortcuts to saving your cash:

- Don't buy too much in the beginning. Yes, it's very tempting, but babies actually need very little aside from the most basic equipment. If they have somewhere safe and comfy to sleep, and some basic clothes and nappies, they are fine. What they need most is you – not the latest electronic gizmo. "If in doubt, don't buy it," says Paul, father of Joshua, eight, Arthur, five, and Mabel, three. "What we realised with Arthur and Mabel, but not with Josh, is that you can actually shop for things after the birth if you need to. If you change your mind on something and decide you really do need it, you can get it. Life doesn't end when the baby arrives – even if you've had a Caesarean, you can buy online."

- On the other hand, if you find something that is an absolute lifeline or your baby adores, consider buying duplicates for grandparents' houses. "A little extra expense is worth not having to mimic a travelling circus every time you pay them a visit," says Mark, father of Jack, two.
- "We bought a chest of drawers instead of a changing table," says Jake, father of Milly, one. "It cost about a third less. We decorated it ourselves – it looks far more individual. And actually, most of the time we use a changing mat on the floor because it's easier and safer. Don't buy things just because they have a 'baby' label on them – look for alternatives."
- "We also used a normal rucksack instead of one of those expensive changing bags," says Jake. "We put in a separate little insulated bottle carrier for the bottles. Marianne didn't mind it, and I was far happier carrying it than some fancy bag that looks like a handbag."
- Remember your baby will grow – quickly. Don't buy too many tiny clothes. Some babies are out of the newborn sizes within a week or two. And don't stockpile small disposable nappies – you will soon need to go up a size.

- Consider splitting the cost of major items which you only need for a few months. If you have a friend whose baby is due a while before or after yours, you can get twice the value at half the cost. Prams and Moses baskets are ideal for this.

- Don't assume that a product with myriad impressive-sounding features will be better than a simpler one – or safer for your child. We had a fairly expensive baby monitor for Evie, which had a temperature alarm on it which sounded if the room temperature went above the 'ideal' range. It was a very hot summer, which meant that nowhere in the entire house fell into that 'ideal' range, not even with the aid of fans, open windows and a lot of nervous fanning from me. So every time we left the room, the alarm sounded. There was nothing to allow you to turn this feature off. In the end, we had to turn the entire monitor off … and then went out and bought a much cheaper version with no temperature alarm.

- Consider a ruthless clear-out of older items once your child has grown out of them – especially if you've finished expanding your family. You could recoup some of the cost by selling them in an online auction. "We sold one of those expensive playpens with a tent on top online," says David, father of Ben, four. "Ben only used it once or twice, he really hated being in it. But with the money we got back, we bought him a new trike."

- Catalogue showrooms, where you select the item from a catalogue and collect it yourself, are good value if you've done your research and know exactly what you want.

- You can hire things you will only use for a short time, such as baby swings and beach cabanas, buggies and larger items. The Baby Equipment Hirers Association has details of local companies. Find it at **www.beha.co.uk**. A couple of recommended ones are **www.tots2go.com** and **www.kidsstuffrentals.co.uk**.

Some people swear by going second-hand. There's lots of nearly new gear about – try charity shops, internet sites, and events organised by the National Childbirth Trust, not to mention family and friends.

top tips

But if you go this route, remember that safety is the key. Second-hand expert Anji, mother of Callum, three, advises:

- Look at the quality of the equipment. Touch surfaces which your baby will touch. If they are rough or sharp, don't buy.
- Be extra careful with hinges, springs and moving parts. These are the places most likely to trap or pinch your baby's fingers and toes.
- If there are small parts, straps or coverings, make sure they can still be fastened properly.
- If it needs to be assembled, make sure it still has its manufacturer's instructions with it. Don't guess and take a chance.
- If it is a piece of equipment directly intended to guarantee the safety of your child, like a car seat, don't take a chance. These are the things to buy new.

Top gear

So, having given yourself a stern talking-to about not over-buying, what exactly are the best things parents recommend?

- "The best thing I have discovered this time is a pop-up travel cot," says Helen, mother of Billy, four, Jeorgy, two, and, recently, baby Dylan. "We took it in our suitcase when we went away. It has a hood, a mosquito net and folds up with a handle like a handbag. He slept through the night in it, and we could also take it to the pool or the beach so he could have a kick or a sleep. One of the worst things about young babies on holiday is that the floors are always tiles, so there is never anywhere to sit them except in a buggy."
- "My friend Vicky bought a grinder for £8 which she uses to purée food for her six month old," says Helen. "It means less money on jars, and fresher food."
- "Another friend, Sarah, takes her Bumbo seat with her everywhere," adds Helen. "She says it's portable, light, and she can feed her nine month old in it, or sit him in it to watch her other son at swimming lessons."
- "I used a nappy laundry service with Olivia," says Victoria, whose daughter is now three. "They delivered freshly washed nappies every week – bliss! It was very expensive though. But I thought it was worth it, to preserve my sanity and to avoid using disposables."
- "If you want to avoid a double buggy, you can get a pram

with a toddler seat on top," says Helen. "It clips on and off easily, and the pram is suitable from birth. Billy, who was two, still needed a bit more of a ride when Jeorgy arrived than a buggy board would have given, so it was perfect. And now he's older, I'm going to put Billy on a buggy board, Jeorgy on the seat and Dylan in the pram, and get all three on it."

- Baby slings are one of those products that inspire debate. Nikki, childminder and mother of George, four, couldn't stand hers. Lisa, mother of Fionn, two, loved the idea. "You can get on and off buses, walk around town, get in and out of shops easily, and have both hands free to try products," says Lisa. "You can even breastfeed in it, with a bit of practice. And it gets you fit."

- "Instead of a Moses basket, buy a crib," says Helen. "The cribs last for six months, compared to about three for the baskets. And the Moses baskets seem a bit flimsy when the babies grow a bit." Nikki disagrees: "We hardly used our wooden cradle at all," she says. "It does last a little longer but it's far more difficult to move about the house or take on visits."

- "The SkipHop changing bag is expensive but great," says Helen. "It has special straps to attach it to a single buggy, plus a shoulder strap to use normally, so you're not always altering the straps to stop it dragging in the mud."

- "Don't waste money on a manual breast pump," adds Helen. "The electric ones are more expensive, but they work."

- "A portable potty is great when you're potty training," says Nikki. "It folds flat when it's not in use. And to save money on the expensive refills, I bought nappy bags and used sanitary towels to soak up the wee."
- The right gear is even more essential when you have twins. Jane, mother of Ethan and Hannah, two, has a few favourites. "The side-by-side double buggies are better than the 'one in front, one behind' ones as the babies can see each other and you easily, and they're also easier if you need to give them both a bottle feed when you're out," she says. "Door bouncers are good for occupying one twin while you feed the other during the day. And bath seats that secure your baby so you don't need to hold them in the bath are good. Buy two and be hands-free to soap each baby in turn. Or just bath one baby while the other is in a bouncer or play nest next to you."
- Georgia, mother of twins Holly and Callum, one, swears by the electronic swing. "Get one of these for your own sanity," she says. "It means you can keep one baby happy if you need to comfort the other. In fact, I loved the swing I borrowed so much, I went out and bought another so they had one each. Also, I used a playpen with a padded floor to lay them to sleep together for naps in the day. It was neater than two bouncy chairs, and meant nobody could tread on them or trip over them."

top tips

As for the products which are firmly on the sneaky parents' blacklist:

- "Baby baths are a total waste of time," says Helen. "After you use them a couple of times, you switch to the main bath – your first baby loves being in the water with you, and if you have two you end up putting them in together." Most parents seemed to agree on this one – and I would add that for a mother with a Caesarean scar, lifting a full baby bath to empty it is not an easy task. One person I know even admitted to converting theirs to an excellent party chiller filled with ice for wine and beer.
- "Spending a lot of money on a pram with a removable carry cot part which you can use as a car seat across the back seat is a waste of money," says Nikki. You can only use it for such a short time, and if you have an older child's car seat in the back too, it won't fit."

And last but not least – the nappy bin. This alert came from several sources, but Nikki sums it up well: "Don't get one – they're useless, and smell disgusting." Some disagree, especially those living in flats with no easily accessible outside bin. But – you have been warned.

To finish, I would say that if you're desperate for an item, go with your gut feeling because different things appeal to different people. But do be aware that, as a parent, you have joined a group of people much loved by marketing men and people trying to sell you things you never even realised existed. So use your head, at least sometimes.

And my personal worst buy ever? It was a gadget that ran off the car cigarette lighter that was supposed to heat up and warm bottles of milk. Very handy, I imagine, should you ever need to warm a bottle of milk while stranded in a car in the middle of a barren land. Which I never did. I think I had visions of being a kind of female, intrepid Yummy Mummy version of explorer Ray Mears. They saw me coming …

CHAPTER 16

Holidays

Kids' clubs and rainy UK breaks – is there life beyond the typical family holiday?

My husband and his sisters were fortunate enough to be taken on family holidays to Disney World in Florida when they were young. They would also, some years, take a UK break at a child friendly holiday camp on the south coast.

He can still remember his parents' wry resignation when, upon being asked by teachers and friends in the autumn what had been the best, most exciting thing they had done that summer, the children replied unanimously: "Going to Hayling Island". For them, the simple pleasures of being able to join the activity clubs and go to the evening 'entertainment' at Hayling was far more memorable than all the magic and thrills that Disney could muster.

This simple truth is something that dawns on most parents within a short time of their first child being born. The days of trekking through the wilds of Borneo, or traversing Indonesia with little more than a sarong and a toothbrush, seem to fade rapidly out of view. Surely, once you have children, it's tour reps, kids' clubs and ball pools all the way?

Now, there are two approaches to this state of affairs.

Either you can give in gracefully and accept that, while it might not be to your taste, joining the bucket and spade brigade at a child friendly resort for a few years makes life a darned sight easier when it comes to entertaining small people and getting some semblance of a break yourself.

Or, you can decide that a more adventurous, intrepid approach where baby comes too – after all, they do have children in Mongolia – will both satisfy your own cravings for the exotic and give your child a wonderfully broad and adaptable outlook on the world at a young age.

There are plenty of tips for both approaches. Please note, though, that sneaky shortcuts relating to the actual 'getting there' side of holidays – car journeys, flights etc – are in the Travel chapter.

Bucket and spade

So, let's start with general tips for your average family friendly holiday. By this, I mean your typical family destinations, such as British beaches, holiday camps here and abroad, campsites, and amusement parks:

- "First of all, be realistic," advises Paul, father of Joshua, eight, Arthur, five, and Mabel, three. "Kids like things like beaches, trains, rides and aquariums. They do not like long car journeys and guided trips around historical monuments. You can try to force them into it, but we've always found that we've had a much nicer holiday all round when we've given the 'customers' what they want."

- Also, be wary of that term "family friendly". It's very vague. Does a two year old want or need the same things as an eight year old or a teenager? Forget such labels slapped on by holiday companies and use your own good sense. Consider the journey time, the facilities, your own child's likes and dislikes, and the cultural attitudes of the country you are considering. Do you want to dine out regularly with your child? Then make sure it's a country like Spain or Italy where children are welcomed in restaurants.
- "Don't assume 'easy' has to mean 'in this country'," says Paul. "Actually, we've found long drives to Cornwall to be harder than a short flight to Spain or the Balearics. And kids find planes, airports and taxis exciting and diverting, whereas the car is just the same boring old car they travel in at home."
- Know your child. If they are clingy, will they really be happy to saunter off to the crèche or kids' club each day on their own?
- Consider taking your own nanny… or if that's not an option, your own relative. "I take my mother with us sometimes," says Nikki, mother of George, four. "It makes all the difference." But make sure you've discussed beforehand exactly how much help they will be willing to offer.
- "If you're going to be travelling late, or just eating out past bedtime, put small children in their pyjamas," says Jane, mother of Ned, two. "We often put Ned in a travel sleep-

ing bag, and just switch him from car or buggy into bed with no fuss when we get back to our villa."

- Conversely, put them to bed in their clothes – a good option if they fall asleep dressed.
- "If you're booking in a campsite or a resort with entertainment, ask when you book exactly where your room or pitch is," says Richard, father of Emily, two. "We had terrible trouble getting Emily off to sleep because we were right near a square with a live cabaret and disco most evenings. In the end, they managed to move us further away, but I wish we'd checked first."
- Consider going out of season. Facilities are emptier, queues for attractions are shorter. If you're going somewhere like Center Parcs where most people check in and out on the same days, try booking your activities such as golf, crazy golf or sauna treatments on those days – everyone else will be busy packing and unpacking, and you'll have the place to yourselves.
- Think in advance how you will actually structure the sleeping arrangements. If your child goes off to sleep by 7pm, and you don't want babysitters, how will you pass the rest of the evening? We usually go self-catering and make sure there is an outside space for us to sit with a bottle of wine and a baby monitor (remember the adapter) for this reason. One friend, Caron, remembers hiding with her husband in a walk-in wardrobe in the dark in a vain attempt to get her son Tom to settle down to sleep in a rather small shared hotel room. When they finally

emerged, they spent the rest of the night reading silently and whispering to each other so as not to wake him up. Another friend, Jackie, always books rooms with a sea view so that she and her husband Peter can soak up the sun on the balcony while their daughter Esme takes a nap.

- Don't overstretch yourselves. A fortnight might seem attractive – even essential – when you're booking, but a short but sweet holiday is often better than a longer stay when you're running around after small children. "I always prefer 10 days to two weeks," says Nikki, mother of George. "A week never seems long enough. As soon as you're starting to relax, it's time to come home – but 14 nights leaves me exhausted."
- "Go back to the sort of places you avoid when you're a couple – family friendly hotels are great," says Helen, mother of Billy, four, Jeorgy, two, and baby Dylan. "Even a baby pool makes a huge difference."
- "The other option I think works really well is a villa with another family," says Helen. "The kids have each other to play with and spend time entertaining themselves so you can have a rest."

Useful things to take:

- Rubber door-stops: "We use them to prop open the internal doors in the villa," says Rob, father of Chloe, four.
- A small spray bottle (you can buy them empty in Boots or other chemist shops) filled with dilute soap solution. "We use them for Chloe because she hates having her hands

washed, especially in loos where they have noisy hand driers." says Rob. "You can also fill them with dilute disinfectant solution for spraying on the loo seat itself."

- Small toys. "We put a couple of favourite toys in a small rucksack which George carries himself," says Nikki. "It keeps him entertained, and makes him feel grown up."
- Back-up supplies. "One time, Olivia's suitcase got delayed in transit," says Piers, whose daughter is three. "It had all her nappies, clothes and toys in it – including her 'essential' cuddly toy for sleeping. It was a nightmare. Now, we share essential stuff between all our bags in case one gets lost."
- Security stuff. "I always label Tom properly, in the time honoured 'Please look after this bear' manner," says Caron. "I use IdentiKids wristbands. I write his name and my mobile number clearly on the band, and he wears it from the time we get to the airport until we get back home at the end of the holiday. When we get to our resort, I add the room number or villa name. The pens are indelible and survive swimming pools with just a few touch-ups from time to time. But be sure you've got your mobile set up to use abroad."
- If the thought of lugging all that gear across continents is making you feel faint, consider ordering it in advance. "We're going to Canada this year," says Nic, mother of Liam, four, and Kieran, eight months. "I found a great website, **www.onetinysuitcase.ca**, where you can get a local person to buy essentials in advance for you. When we arrived at our hotel, food, nappies and formula for two

> weeks were waiting for us at reception. I have since discovered that there are companies which do the same in other countries, including Spain. You can even arrange to hire big items such as car seats, travel cots, buggies and toys. So no carrying."

Food and drink

What puts some families off travelling abroad is the food and drink issue. But actually, you'd be amazed at which different 'specialities' can appeal to small children. Often, they'll try things in a new, exciting environment that they'd pick at in disgust at home. On a recent trip to France, we were astonished when Evie demanded her own bowl of mussels and calmly set about picking each one neatly from its shell and devouring them with gusto. This, from a child whose previous adventures with fish extended mainly to the kind offered by Captain Birds Eye.

So give it a go – and remember, small amounts of finger food are often more successful than presenting your sceptical three year old with a loaded plate of something unidentifiable. A quick rundown of successful snacks garnered from sneaky parents includes tapas, tortilla, meatballs and paella in Spain; moussaka and souvlaki (skewered meat) in Greece; croque monsieur and sausages in France; noodles in Thailand; grilled chicken or fresh fish and chips in Corsica or Greece or Portugal; fish cutters (breaded fish in a bun) and rice in the Caribbean.

As for small babies, they are at their most adaptable if they are still breastfeeding – no worries about bacteria or contaminated food. Just take a sling, a hat and some sunblock and you're off – all food and drink is on tap.

And for older children, a positive attitude can work wonders. "Just remember, if you get stressed about what they're eating, they won't eat," says Paul. "If they survive on bread and cheese and ice cream for a week, it's not the end of the world. Just make sure they drink plenty – take bottled water or a Thermos of boiled water everywhere. And if you can't get hold of water, try a brand-name fizzy drink – you might not give it to them at home, but the drinks are bottled under strict regulations so they are a safe stopgap."

Outward bound

Finally, what if you've decided that, easy or not, there just has to be life beyond the 'child friendly' option? Do you have to be an intrepid adventurer to take your children beyond the holiday frontiers of Spain and Greece? Here are a few tips from people who think not.

"When children are young is just the right time to try new things with them," says Lisa, mother of Fionn, two. "They haven't made up their minds that it's anything odd." Lisa and husband James are planning a holiday to Yosemite and Sequoia National Parks in the USA. "We're keen walkers, so we're going to fly to San Francisco, pick up a pre-booked 4x4, and then drive across to the parks where we can hike with Fionn in a backpack," says Lisa. "We have pre-booked a few cabins and will stay at those along the way, but we're also leaving a lot of it loose."

Helen agrees that some longer-haul options are worth trying, even with young ones. "We went to Florida last year when we had two children, aged three and nearly one," says Helen. "We went with another family. We were worried that perhaps our two were too young, but actually it was a brilliant age because at that age they still believe it really is the real Winnie the Pooh and Snow White. They loved it."

Nic and Hugh are also veterans of the more exotic family holiday. They loved to travel before they had children and saw no reason to stop after the arrival of Liam and Kieran. When Liam was a young toddler they travelled to Japan. "It was amazing," says Nic. "Liam only slept briefly on the 12-hour flight, but that seemed to help him adjust to the time difference, which he dealt with better than we did. He'd never slept in a bed before, but we put the bed up against the wall and put pillows under the mattress so it slanted towards the wall to stop him falling out.

"Milk was initially a problem because he didn't like the taste but we bought him cartons of flavoured milk which they sold in a vending machine in our Tokyo hotel. He loved going to buy it. When we couldn't get that, he had yoghurt drinks. Our hotel had a music room, a soft play area, and outdoor play area and an art room – but we didn't use them much because he would get as excited about sightseeing as we were. The attention he got from the Japanese probably had something to do with it – he's blond, and wherever we went people were giving him presents and taking his photo.

"As for eating, the Japanese seem to like Italian food, so we'd alternate. Liam ate pasta and Japanese rice, and we told him noodles were pasta so he ate those.

"We travelled around on the Bullet train, and once we used Liam for an excellent photo opportunity. At the train station a group of Geishas came along with their chaperone. I would have been too shy to take their photo, but I walked up with Liam and they were happy to pose with him. In years to come, he will be able to proudly show off a photo of himself surrounded by Geisha girls."

She admits to just one challenge: "The only problem we had was nappies – Japanese children are much smaller, and we had to make do with nappies that were too small. One day I thought I'd cracked it and found a larger size, only to discover through sign language that I was trying to buy incontinence knickers."

It seems that a relaxed, can-do attitude can be the best of all sneaky tips if you're thinking of pushing the boundaries. If you're the kind of person, like me, who can't get as far as Mallorca without six suitcases full of all kinds of 'just in case' supplies, then maybe you should wait until your children are older. But if you have the ability to wing it and adapt, then there's no doubt your children will get the experience of a lifetime.

This year, Nic and Hugh are off on a trip round Canada. "We're flying in and out of Calgary and have hired a motor home to travel around in," Nic says. "We have an idea of a possible itinerary but no concrete plans. We'll get to explore national parks such as Banff and Jasper. I'm not entirely sure where Kieran will sleep yet – there'll be no room for a crib or carrycot – but we'll just make him a makeshift bed somewhere snug. It will be fine."

And it will. Because she will make sure it is. I am trying, very hard, to follow her example. I might even leave behind the kitchen sink on our next trip to Mallorca.

CHAPTER 17

Flying the nest

Playgroups, pre–schools and nursery school – how to let them go

So you've battled your way through sleeping and feeding disasters, braved potty training, dealt with tantrums and travel traumas and even managed to transport your child overseas without chartering a private plane just for the baby equipment.

Now it's time to send them to pre-school for a few hours a week, and you'd think you would be hanging out the banners in exhausted celebration.

You'd think. But that weird thing that happens in parents' brains kicks in – and, when it actually comes to sending our little ones out into the world on their own for the first time, most of us turn into quivering jellies of guilt and nerves.

Here is not the place to go into too much detail regarding all the variations of 'pre-school' available. In a nutshell, most areas offer some form of pre-schooling from around the age of two and a half or just after that.

Some concentrate on a more play-oriented environment for the first year and then switch children to a slightly more formal kindergarten or nursery environment for the year which precedes entry into the reception class at primary school. Other areas keep the children in the same environment right through from two until five. Some use labels such as Playgroup followed by Nursery, others describe it as Nursery followed by Kindergarten. Some do mornings only, some afternoons.

There's actually no law that says you have to send your child to any kind of pre-school or nursery. As long as they're in school by the age of five, that's fine. But most parents recognise that taking a few steps away from the home environment before that can be a very positive, confidence-building, self-affirming thing for a toddler, not to mention a lifeline for an overstretched parent with possibly other, smaller, demanding siblings still at home, or indeed a job to go to.

So we gird our loins and get ready to nudge our babies gently out of the nest. But it's hard. Probably even harder for us than it is for them. So how can we ease the way as they take those first steps of freedom?

Getting ready

Build up to their first day by talking about it a few weeks beforehand (not too far in advance, because time goes slowly at that age). Also:

- Think 'strength in numbers'. Local establishments will probably have more familiar faces as local children join at the same time. "It really helped that George went to mother and toddler group in the same village as playgroup," says Nikki, mother of George, four, and also a very in-demand childminder in the same village. "The children in the village sort of 'go up through the ranks' and can see the older children doing these things before them. They realise it's going to be their turn one day so it makes it easier for them. George is at Nursery now. He said to me today: 'I don't like nursery any more, I just can't wait to go to reception.'"

- Arrange a play date with another child who will be attending the same pre-school. Get their parents to give some sneaky positive reinforcement, and do the same with their child. "Jackie did this with Esme," says Peter, whose daughter started pre-school last year. "She made it seem like an adventure they were going on together. So Esme had a little friend which boosted her confidence for the first few weeks. Now, they've both branched off a bit as they've got more confident."
- When it's time to go on that first day, don't dither. Go in with purpose, perhaps visit the toilets with them, help them find their seat, and leave. Cry outside if you have to – I did – but only when you're out of sight.
- Let your child help pack their own bag – with spare clothes, underwear etc – in the morning. "It helps them feel grown up, but it also means that they can identify their own stuff more easily during the day," says Jackie. Needless to say, label everything.
- You could consider letting them take a 'transitional object' such as a favourite cuddly toy to comfort themselves with.

However, some pre-schools dislike this as they have too many treasured objects either going astray or being fought over. We took this opportunity to have Evie's Blue Bear stay at home while she was busy being a 'big girl at school'. He waits either by the front door or in her car seat for her to come home.

Loosening the apron strings

However well you prepare them – and you – for the big day, you will inevitably feel something of a wobble when it actually comes to letting them go.

But you don't want to cramp their style – so get sneaky. Become a furtive peeker-through-windows, if the layout of your pre-school premises allows it, or seek some 'inside information' from a willing – and they are always willing – member of staff. Because practically all children who create a fuss when you leave will, often within seconds of you disappearing from sight, calm instantly and become absorbed in the children, chatter and toys around them.

So, check up on them. Watch them when they think you're not there. Get mini 'reports' from the staff: how long did they take to calm down? Some good pre-schools even offer to call new parents half an hour after dropping-off time to reassure them that all is well.

Just one thing: some children do a kind of 'double bluff' and start nursery fantastically well, only to regress to clingy, upset behaviour anything from a couple of days to a couple of weeks later. This is because they've suddenly realised that this is not some temporary diversion but an ongoing arrangement, and they're not sure that's quite what they signed up to. Surf it – it invariably passes after a few days.

Nikki says: "George was pretty good at starting playgroup. Because of the childminding, he already knew some of the children there and had been with me to drop them off. He was good for the first week and then I think it hit home that when I left, he had to stay. So for the second week it was horrendous at drop-off time.

"But let me just say, from a childminder's point of view, it's all just show for the mummy. All the children I take did it for a while, but as soon as the door is shut behind them and mummy is gone, they are fine. I spoke to the playgroup leader and she said it's best to walk out and leave them, as however hard it is leaving your screaming darling behind, the longer you stay the worse it is for you and for them."

Lyn, mother of Jack, seven, and also a playgroup staff member, agrees. "They can be a real barrel load of monkeys when it comes to parents leaving. It's all a big show just for you. Once you're out of sight, invariably they settle down, even on those first few days."

It's the process of separating from you that they find hard. Once you've gone, it's fine. Doing the whole 'I'll stay just a few minutes then' process is actually, unwittingly, the cruellest thing you can do. It's actually far kinder, if harder for you, to hand them over, give them a kiss, say goodbye (while they scream) and just go.

Lyn also suggests telling teachers what your child's favourite 'thing of the moment' is – fairies, or fire engines, or dinosaurs, or fluffy rabbits. "Then the staff have some 'inside information' when it comes to distracting them if they get upset," she says.

For parents of twins worried that their children may be too dependent on each other, or may not be seen as individuals by teachers or peers, Jane, mother of Ethan and Hannah, two, says: "This is more of an issue for identical twins, but I'd suggest trying doing the odd day when only one of the twins is at pre-school and the other at home."

Getting involved

Once your child is established at pre-school, it's easy to feel that they have suddenly embarked on a whole area of life to which you have no access or input. This can be very unsettling to parents who have been used to controlling and shaping every last spit and cough of their precious baby's existence.

But you don't need to feel cut out. In fact, the more you get stuck in there and involved with your child's pre-school experience, the better:

- Talk to the pre-school leader and teachers and find out as much information as you can about the routines and experiences your child will encounter. Good pre-schools will be only too keen to show you examples of other children's work, the curriculum and activities. "I found this very helpful when Esme started," says Jackie. "Because I'd had a good chat with her playgroup leader, I could answer all her questions about when snack time was, what happened if she needed help in the loo, when she would get to play outside and lots of other stuff. It helped me reassure her."

- Find out what areas or themes will be covered that term. Good pre-schools may send a newsletter outlining this. If they are studying transport, or life cycles, or weather, you can play along at home and help your child apply this to the outside world.
- Be nice to the teachers. Many pre-schools rely on parent help either on committees or just on an ad hoc basis. It may sound cynical but if you're one of the ones getting stuck in at the fete, running a stall or baking cakes or helping to put up marquees, you can be sure you'll pick up sooner whether or not your child is a happy customer.

Clear and simple

Think, too, how you can make the everyday practicalities of pre-school easier for your child. Simple tasks like pulling up a pair of trousers, or finding a coat, can be monumental for them. Bigger stuff like how to share toys and make friends is what pre-school is all about – but if you can help with the small stuff, chances are they'll have a better shot at mastering the big things and having fun too.

top tips

Good shortcuts include:

- Use visual aids. Evie's pre-school uses a picture to go with her name on labels – she has an elephant because it starts with the same letter as her name. When she arrives each day, she finds her name tag and hangs it on a little wooden tree, which shows which children are in that day. The same symbol and name are on a label to show where she should sit. Parents can adapt this idea – to small children, all name tapes look the same, so draw a little symbol next to their name which they can recognise, such as a smiley face, or a star or a butterfly.
- If your child wants – and is allowed – to take a favourite cuddly toy, make sure it is labelled clearly. "Emily was desperate to take her 'Binty'," says Richard. "But Jill and I were petrified she'd lose it because she only sleeps if she can cuddle it. So Jill sewed on one of those little identity tags you get for cats and dogs, engraved with our phone number and the words 'Emily's Binty'. Emily loved it, and if she loses it, we might stand some chance of getting it back."
- Forget clothes with lots of buttons and fiddly belts. "Go elasticated," says Jackie. "And use shoes with Velcro fastenings."

By the way, once your child starts pre-school, it is only fair to warn you that mums and dads, too, enter a new realm: that of the competitive parent. You thought toddler group was bad enough, with comparisons of how adept your little one was at grabbing the most chocolate biscuits or making the best Play-Doh monsters? It gets worse.

The thing is, every parent believes that their child is, of course, not only the most charming but also the most intelligent, caring, creative and popular child in their class. Unfortunately we can't all always be right. And the day comes when you are presented with the fact that your child has done something unspeakable – weed in the Wendy house, or imprinted another child with a perfect set of teeth marks, or refused to join in 'What's the Time Mister Wolf?' with a protest that threatened to require the presence of the local police.

Your first instinct will be to deny, and then to defend. My child? No way. Absolutely not. And even if they did, they must have been led into it, coerced by the class bad boy.

The thing is, nobody's child is perfect. If they were, they'd be a bit creepy. They're there to learn. So believe the staff if they tell you that your child's done something undesirable. Take it on board, talk to your child at home, and be a team with your pre-school. Trust them – they've seen and done it all before.

And when your baby takes part in their first nativity, or brings home their first attempt at a crudely made Father's Day card, or recites a rhyme you didn't teach them, you'll cry even more than you did the day they set off without you. Only this time, they'll probably raise their eyes to the heavens and wail that eternal refrain that tells you your child is growing up: "Oh, Mu–uuumm!"

CHAPTER 18

You

Fitting 'me time' into your child's social diary; reclaiming your wobbly bits

This was a hard chapter to research. The reason? Sorry to hit you in the face with this, but most of the parents I talked to felt that they were a little lacking on the 'me time' tips. It's just that they were ... well, a little too tied up with their children to have had much practice.

"Tips on pampering and getting away?" says Helen, mother of three boys under five. "I have to say I don't have much time for that." This was said via email, and if there were an emoticon available to suggest a feeling of grim black humour, Helen would have used it.

This is also a chapter which unavoidably focuses rather more on the mother than the father. Most of the book will hopefully be equally useful whichever parent you happen to be. This one, while recognising that fathers undergo their own tiredness/self-esteem/time management issues, aims to be useful to both but inevitably sometimes refers to the mother, especially if we're talking physical issues. But even then, it should provide some useful tips which dads can help with, or at least an insight into the murky world of new maternal angst.

So, having said that, the whole idea of 'you' becomes irrevocably mutated once you have a child. That's not to say you can't find yourself again – it's just that you might have to accept that, in at least a minor and very probably a major way, that 'you' has altered. And you're not going to come to terms with that overnight.

My best tip is to think small. Don't be imagining dramatic returns to form in the manner of a Hollywood star with a personal chef, nanny and oversized bank account. Unless you are 20 or under, with muscles ready to snap back into action the second you leave the hospital, that's not going to happen.

What does work, though, is making tiny changes which add up to a much happier you. Five minutes here and there. A meal out. A manicure. A half-hour bath, with no interruptions … these can make all the difference. Not rocket science, admittedly, but believe me, when you're so tired you can barely contemplate getting dressed before you leave the house, these can be major achievements.

Beating baby blues

The best place to start regarding some sneaky 'me time' shortcuts is probably the early days, when you first come home with the baby:

- Steel yourself for chaos and fatigue, and don't beat yourself up if the washing-up is not done/the plants have died/you look like an extra from The Munsters/there's sick down the baby's best sleep suit. "I'd say just accept that the first six weeks will be a whirlwind, and it'll all settle down after that," says Helen, mother of Billy, four, Jeorgy, two, and baby Dylan.

- "Don't be proud," says Nikki, childminder and mother of George, four. "Take up any offers of help. Grab every five minutes when you can." You could even ask for a day of someone's time instead of a baby gift.
- "A month before you're due, cook double of everything and freeze half," says Nikki. "Do it with grown-up portions and for any existing children. I found this a lifesaver. After George was born, I had a month's worth of meals just waiting – I'd defrost them and put them with fresh vegetables. Cooking nutritious food is the last thing you want to do from scratch when you arrive home with a screaming baby."
- Nikki adds: "Ask friends to come to visit, but ask them to bring lunch with them – close friends are only too happy to do this. That way, you get the company but no work."
- "I really struggled with breastfeeding," remembers Marianne, mother of Milly, one. "I felt like a complete failure, and very alone. But I asked my health visitor to put me in touch with other mothers who were finding it hard, and we actually started to meet up for coffee and help each other through. It was a real lifeline at an awful time."
- Rely on your partner if you can. If you're breastfeeding, fathers can often feel that there's little for them to do. But they can still change nappies, feed expressed milk, help

with housework, distract an older sibling, wind the baby after a feed, take the baby out for a walk while you sleep … and just be there in the middle of the night when it's tough. I remember that Lewis's night-time walks along the landing singing endless repeats of Old MacDonald were a wonderful, if sleepy, bonding experience for him and quite possibly also the thing that stopped me throwing myself out of the bedroom window when she wouldn't sleep.

- Remember, the early days are a time when you should be concentrating on the tiny microcosm of a world that is you and your baby. Forget chores and errands – this is the one time of your life that people will, truly, understand and not comment snidely behind your back. If you feel you must do a few household chores, try to adapt them to make them as easy as possible. For instance, buy ready-to-go cleaning wipes to give the bathroom sink a quick spruce up, rather than scrubbing away with your normal detergent. "If you've had a Caesarean, put the ironing board on the very lowest height setting," says Nikki. "That way, you can sit on the sofa and iron a few bits without standing or straining your scar."

The thing that will keep you sane in the early days is to include tiny, sporadic amounts of the activities you used to enjoy. "It took me a while to realise that, with a small baby, they just want your presence – they don't need your undivided attention the way that older ones do," says Marianne. "So you can be with them, but also maybe read a chapter of a book, or knit, or write a journal. They're just as happy watching you relax with a hobby as they would be watching you do the washing-up. And a friend told me to make the most of that before they start demanding that you help them with a jigsaw or build a rocket for Buzz Lightyear."

top tips

Other 'young baby' tips:

- "Reclaim your arms," advises Anji, mother of Callum, three. "When Callum was tiny, I reckon I spent about half my time holding him and the other half thinking of safe places I could put him down. One thing I used to do when I'd run out of ideas was take a bath with him on my chest. Yes, I was still holding him, but he loved the sensation of the water, and I got a good soak."
- "Also, stay in pyjamas for at least the first week," says Anji. "They're comfortable, and they're a good signal that when visitors arrive unannounced – which they always do – you're not up to a long visit."
- Find ways to keep yourself calm and entertained during night-time feeds. "Amy found those night feeds so boring," says Mark, father of Jack. "Then I started renting some DVDs for her of silly comedy movies, and she would watch them while she fed Jack on the sofa. The comedies worked best because they made her laugh through her tiredness, kept her spirits up and didn't need a lot of concentration." The same goes for radio. "I fed mine in the bedroom and didn't have a TV, so I listened to CDs of Radio 4 comedies such as *I'm Sorry, I Haven't A Clue*," says Roni, mother of Jack, now 10, Ned, eight, and Hal, five. "It certainly kept me jolly despite no sleep."

- "Don't get your baby too used to being held all the time," says Melanie, mother of Joshua, eight, Arthur, five, and Mabel, three. "As soon as they've finished eating, put them in a safe place with toys, like a play mat or bouncy seat. This is their most contented time, and it will teach them to be happy on their own for small amounts of time. When you've got older children, this is essential – all the usual tips for parents of newborns seem to be aimed at first-timers, but when you've got toddlers tearing around armed with glue, glitter and lots of energy, you have to find different strategies."

Caroline, mother of Heather, four, and Murray, one, agrees that nothing prepares you for baby number two … or more. "I didn't appreciate the value of having just one child," she recalls. "Now, even with 'only' two children, I find I have practically zero time for me. I don't work officially, so I'm seen by my husband and other mums as 'not doing anything'. They think I must have plenty of free time. But I'm a 'can't say no' person, and have ended up on every committee going, with a volunteer job too. Oh yes, and being a mum."

Caroline remembers joining a private leisure club when Murray was very young. "I just needed to get away from the crying, so I'd go for a swim in the evening when I nearly always had the big swimming pool to myself," she says. "The novelty wore off after about six months, but it was a great escape."

She warns, though, against being too creative with 'getting away from it' ideas during those first few months of muddle-headedness. "It became a bit of a mission to find some peace," she laughs. "To get both children to go off to sleep, I would drive around the surrounding area, wait until they had both dropped off, then pull into a quiet spot overlooking the river, get my book out and relax. After about six months of doing this, I finally noticed one day that all the other people pulled over into this beauty spot were men, and were getting out of their cars and disappearing into the bushes. It transpired that I was 'relaxing' in a west of Scotland 'dogging' hotspot. I felt so bad."

Rather more suitable locations for relaxation which Caroline recommends are places childless couples go. "I do insist on going to child-free places when I finally get the chance to go out shopping or for lunch on my own," she says. "I hang out in art galleries, or restaurants and coffee shops with lots of stairs. I look for 'difficult to manoeuvre a pram' situations and go and hide there."

Older child strategies

Once your baby is a little bigger, and right through toddlerhood and beyond, there are a few more shortcuts you can employ to give yourself some time.

This is the time to stand back, take a good look at yourself as an individual – and yourselves as a couple – and remember *who you are.*

- Look after yourself physically. Take an hour out to go swimming, or walking, or cycling. Your child will be fine with a grandparent, friend or in a crèche by this age – you do not have to feel guilty for doing something for yourself.

- Remember the things you used to enjoy both alone and with your partner or friends. Rediscover them.
- Buy some new clothes if you can. Put away those pyjamas and tracksuit bottoms.

The one thing new parents are short of is time. This is where you need to adapt how you do things in order to claw back some time for yourself. As with new babies, think short breathing spaces rather than large chunks of time – a drip-drip of bite-size opportunities to refuel yourself mentally. No time for dinner with friends? Meet for a cup of coffee and a bun. Can't go to bed in the daytime? Put the Moses basket downstairs and relax on the sofa with a pillow and a duvet the minute your baby drops off to sleep next to you.

Also, write things down. Plan for 'me time' on your calendar – if it's there in black and white, you're more likely to go through with it, even after a bad day. "The one thing which really works for us is that we have a babysitter who we have booked in advance for the first Friday night of every month," says Helen. "This means that even when we feel too tired to go out, we have to go – which is great, because you always end up having a good time when you make the effort. And it at least means we get out once a month together.

"A friend of mine has a similar arrangement with a friend where every other week they babysit for each other, which again forces them to take time for themselves because the other couple is relying on it too."

Christine, Evie's grandmother, remembers a more complicated babysitting system she was part of with her three children, which works well within a close group of trusted friends or with young parents all living close to each other, for instance on a street or estate. “We had a kind of credit system where we’d keep track of how many nights out or nights babysitting each parent had ‘used’,” she says. “I remember it often seemed more trouble than it was worth, because I felt I really had to tidy up the house – if another woman was coming in, it had to be spotless. I used to spend all day cleaning, wishing I wasn’t going out. But when we got there, we’d really enjoy it.”

Even if you don’t want a babysitter so you can go out of the house, establish a time in the evening by which children are in bed, and you get time to ‘just be’ – without chores. “My aim in life is not to do housework after the children’s bedtime,” says Caroline. “I will do anything to achieve that. I have an unwritten rule that when Daddy stops work, so should I. You need the mental separation from work and children to be refreshed for another day.”

With twins, it’s even more essential to get some help if family, friends or funds allow it. “I’ve had a lady come to me on a Friday since the twins were quite small to iron the children’s clothes, feed them, bathe them, play with them and keep their rooms tidy,” says Jane, mother of Ethan and Hannah, two, and big sister Emily, five. “I don’t think I would have a hair on my head if I had not had this. When they were younger I stayed in the house while she was there, but now as I’ve got braver I venture out to do errands or shopping. And a coffee shop and a magazine do wonders for the system.”

And Georgia, mother of twins Callum and Holly, one, believes that total strangers hold the key to boosting the self-esteem of a new mother of twins. "I remember a woman I'd never seen before in my life shouting to me across a car park in Brentwood 'Congratulations! You got out of the house!'" she laughs. "But my best feelgood tip for mums of twins, particularly if you also have another child, is to go to your local baby clinic with your tribe in tow and sit with all the new mothers who are finding it hard with their first baby. They look at you like you're Superwoman. It boosts you so much to bask in the awe of new mums – you leave thinking 'Yes! I am the best!'"

Mirror image

Throughout all of this, from Day One with a new baby right through the older childhood days, is the issue of your own self-esteem. Yes, there are lots of things you can *do* to help you feel more like yourself. But what about what you *are* – what about, to be blunt, what you *look like*?

Body image and – whisper it – the 'sex thing' are the true unspoken bugbears of early parenthood. They affect both mothers and their partners to a degree which nobody warns you about before you conceive, because probably the truth would be the most effective form of contraception known to man.

But here are the bare facts of it, so to speak: after a baby, your body will not be the same. Ever again. If you're young, super-fit and disciplined, you might get back to a near approximation of what you were before – with a few shifts here, a widening there, a lone stretch mark somewhere else. If you're like most of us, you will be left with bits that hang, bits that have drooped, bits that bulge and bits that appear to have been grafted on to you by the Hammer House of Horror special effects department while you slept.

It can all be very depressing. In the very early days, you're still so much in shock that you actually gave birth to this baby to really take in the damage. At this stage, it's all about just getting through. If you manage to pull on clean clothes and remove yesterday's mascara – congratulations, you applied mascara – then you've done well. So just concentrate on the basics. "A great tip I was told was to use baby products for your own skin," remembers Marianne. "After all, they're geared up to be suitable for the most sensitive skin around. I used baby lotion to keep my hands soft, and baby wipes to take off my make-up. Also, the zinc stuff you use to get rid of nappy rash is great for getting rid of a spot. Just dab a tiny bit on and wait in case you get a reaction before using it again."

One other tip I might add is – if you can and you're close – spend a little time with your mother. No, really. There is nobody on earth like a mother to tell you – and *really believe* – that you are beautiful. My mother is the best at this. And even when you might suspect she is wearing some rather impressive rose-tinted spectacles, it's still nice to hear it, especially from someone who once felt just as awful after your grand entrance into the world.

Eventually, there comes a time when you start to feel a lot more like your old self than you thought possible. The idea of fitting more than your big toe into your pre-pregnancy jeans becomes just – only just – conceivable. You start to look at clothes in shops again, and maybe diet a bit, and dream of being … normal. Attractive. Maybe even … sexy. And the best tip here is: be realistic. You are a mother now. Find a way of being the best 'you' right now, not being the 'you' that you were before. "I'm not sure I have got my body back," laughs Nikki, whose son George is four. "I think I was just a blob since I was born. God, I want to be thin …" Nikki, by the way, is a dab hand at the self–deprecating thing.

And then, of course, there's the issue of getting intimate. The doctors' line on this is usually "Six weeks, madam, and then you may resume 'relations'". Which is just the thing most new mothers do not wish to hear. In fact, the thought of anybody – anybody – coming within three feet of the parts of us which have just been traumatised beyond belief is enough to send many of us running for the hills.

There are lots of books available which go into detail about resuming a sex life after the birth of a child. Most mention starting off slowly, spending time with a partner cuddling and being close before leaping into the sack, and helping yourself to feel sexy by giving yourself time to relax and be pampered rather than by reluctantly fishing out your sexy underwear and doing your best pole dancer impression. Ouch.

If all that fails and you need just a little more time during which to resurrect your libido, I do have one tip from a mother who shall, for the sake of her own personal 'relations', remain nameless: "Tell him your doctor sadly said 'no go' for three more months," she says with a wicked grin. "It's doctor's orders – so it's out of your hands."

Also, remember that dads, too, have a lot of adjusting to do after the birth of a baby. They may have their undercarriages intact, but very often their egos, self-esteem, identities and roles at home have taken something of a battering. Whether you are a mum or a dad, remember, if you can, to talk to each other. As long as you're talking, albeit in a sporadic and sleep-starved fashion, you'll probably be OK.

Finally, remember that the only person who can reclaim you is – you. But sometimes, the best people to help you see who that person is are the people around you. These are the people who love you, who find you gorgeous, who are proud of who you are and what you've done. Listen to them, they're right.

They may also be the people who you meet at the soft play centre, or the postnatal group, or the toddler morning – who don't know you that well yet, but who sure as hell know what it's like to face a body in the mirror which sports not so much a 'muffin' effect over the jeans waistband, but more of an EU food mountain.

The whole point of this book is that the best advice comes from real parents who have done it, seen it and felt it all before – so listen to every last sneaky tip and shortcut you are offered. Use some, discard some, but never forget that there is always a way to make things just a little bit easier. And soon, you'll be the expert yourself. Good luck!

Acknowledgements

This is a book for what I call 'real parents' – and the only way to write one of those is to *talk* to real parents. I am no expert in the traditional sense of the word, but I do feel that all parents are experts when it comes to their own children, and their own tips gained through bitter experience.

I would, then, like to thank the following 'experts' for their invaluable help with this book, and for putting up with my endless requests for the next round of tips.

Evie's NCT group: Nic, Hugh, Liam and Kieran; Caroline, Graham, Heather and Murray; Jess, Colin, Molly and Daisy; Georgia, Ed, Woody, Callum and Holly; Alice, Simon, Sam and Ben; Christine, John, Amie and Jessica; Charlotte, Mark, Eleanor and Jack.

The Much Hadham Mother and Toddler Group, as well as teachers and parents of Evie's friends at the Much Hadham Playgroup and at St Andrew's School.

Many patient Much Hadham friends including: Nikki, Gary and George; Jo, Phil, Archie and Charlotte; Julie, Michael, Michael and Maddie; Laura, Andy and Max; Sandra, Graham, Ben and Toby; Jill, David and Jessica; Lisa, James and Fionn; Caron, Paul and Tom; Jane, Andy, Emily, Ethan and Hannah.

Old friends and assorted work colleagues and acquaintances including: Amy, Mark and Jack; Jackie, Peter and Esme; Mandy, David and Ben; Jill, Richard and Emily; Victoria, Piers and Olivia; Marianne, Jake and Milly; Anji and Callum; Helen, David, Billy, Jeorgy and Dylan; Debbie, Mark, Abbie and Daniel; Richard, Kate, Oliver, Jessica and Emily; Claire, Jon and Sam; Jane, Dan and Ned; Liz, Steve and Lily; Sian, Mark, Joe and Jenny; Melanie, Dave, Joshua, Arthur and Mabel; Jenna, Mark, Daniel, Tom and Rory; Emma, Rob and Chloe; Andrew, Madeleine and Eleanor; Ben, Alison, Joe, Abigail and Lara.

Family, including Maxine, Dave, and Evie's cousins Marnie and Freddy; Estelle; my lovely mother-in-law Christine who, with my very much missed father-in-law Tex, did a fantastic job with my husband and his two sisters; Barb, Mark, Kate and Victoria; Lindsey; my father Tony and stepfather Colin; and my mother Annie who is an inspirational mother and grandmother.

My Uncle Jim, who we lost just a few days before this book was completed. He was the kind of man everybody loved and who knew the importance of family.

Roni (who believed a sleep-starved and time-deprived journalist could actually write a book), her boys Jack, Ned and Hal, and her team at White Ladder Press.

Lastly, my amazing husband Lew who, in the words of my daughter, is "The Best Daddy in the World", and Evie herself, who lights up all our lives.

PS Evie's baby brother Charlie has just made his entrance – watch this space for forthcoming books specialising in sibling warfare.